Testimonials

What readers and the medical community say...

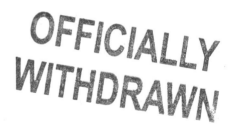

W9-BAH-259

"Chef Dave's cookbooks have been a tremendous help to the weight loss community. As the premier chef for bariatrics, Chef Dave has never failed to wow us with his knowledge, talent and delicious food. ***Ditch Your Diet in 30 Days*** is no different. With recipes that are not only great tasting, but easy to make, this book is a must have for anyone concerned with maintaining a healthy lifestyle."

- Colleen M. Cook
President, Bariatric Support Centers International

"***Ditch Your Diet in 30 Days*** is an awesome tool for people who are serious about weight-loss success and want to enjoy satisfying food."

- Katie Jay, MSW
National Association for Weight Loss Surgery

"***Ditch Your Diet in 30 Days*** is perfect for families who want delicious and nutritionally balanced meals. Chef Dave guides you with a simple to follow meal plan that makes creating healthy meals quick and easy. This is a terrific book for anyone looking to eat healthier and manage his or her weight."

- Rebecca K. Ricard
Publisher, WLS Lifestyles magazine

Ditch Your Diet in 30 Days

90 Easy, Healthy Meals and Snack Recipes for Effective Weight Loss

Chef Dave Fouts
and
Vicki Bovee, M.S., R.D.

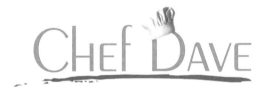

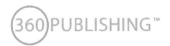

Reno, NV

360° Publishing, LLC.

3495 Lakeside Drive, Suite 205

Reno, Nevada 89509, USA

Visit Chef Dave's website at www.chefdave.org

This publication is designed to provide general information regarding the subject matter covered. The general health and nutritional information provided is intended for informational purposes only. The subject matter is not intended to be a substitute for professional nutritional or medical advice, diagnosis, or treatment. Readers of this subject matter should not rely exclusively on the information provided through this subject matter for their own health needs. All specific medically and nutritionally oriented questions should be presented to your own health care providers.

The author has taken reasonable precautions in the preparation of this subject matter and believes that facts presented are accurate as of the date it was written. The author has followed all guidelines with regard to United States Department of Agriculture and the American Dietary Association guidelines. Both the author and publisher specifically disclaim any liability resulting from the use or application of the information contained in the subject matter and the information is not intended to serve as medical or nutritional advice as it relates to anyone's individual situations.

Further, neither the author nor the publisher make any warranties or representations, express or implied, as to the accuracy or completeness, timeliness, or usefulness of any opinions, advice, services, or other information contained or referenced in this subject matter.

If you purchase this book without a cover, you should be aware that this book may have been stolen property and reported as "unsold and destroyed" to the publisher. In such case, neither the author nor the publisher has received any payment for this "stripped book."

Printed in the United States of America

Publisher's Cataloging-In-Publication Data
(Prepared by The Donohue Group, Inc.)

Fouts, Dave.
    Ditch your diet in 30 days : 90 easy, healthy meals and snakc recipes for
effective weight loss/ Dave Fouts and Vicki Bovee.

              p. ; cm.

    Includes index.
    ISBN: 978-1-934727-21-8

1. Reducing diets--Popular works. 2. Reducing diets--Recipes. 3. Weight loss--Popular works. 4. Nutrition. I. Bovee, Vicki. II. Title.

RM222.2 .F68 2009

613.2/5

ISBN 978-1-934727-21-8

Dedication

This book is dedicated to my family. I am one of five children and my sisters and brothers helped transform me into the person I am today. To Amanda, you helped me grow as a person and never gave up on my crazy ideas. You have given me determination and a drive to accept nothing but the best. To Patrick, your sense of humor and way you look at life has a way of making me laugh even at the most awkward times, giving me humility. To Chip, my baby bro, in constant motion and seeking every corner to live your life and seek your dreams on your terms, you have taught me to see the glass half full. Last but certainly not least, Brittany, we have a bond that is unexplainable. We know what each other is thinking and feeling without saying a word, instinct by the very definition is what I have received from you. I love all of you more than you possibly know and want to thank you for helping to shape me into the husband, dad, son, and brother that I am.

To my mom who was crazy enough to have five children. You are a true inspiration and have always been there to help carry me through the rough times and lift my wings when I'm soaring. I am forever grateful for your courage, kindness, and wisdom.

To my wife Mary, when we first met we only knew that I hated to do laundry and that you hated to cook. It was a match made in heaven. Twelve years later and thousands of loads of laundry and meals, and I'm still amazed in your presence. You are a strong woman, an awesome mother, and I am your biggest fan.

To Noah and Michael, I am the proudest dad on the planet. You are growing up way too fast, and having you two as my sons truly is my biggest accomplishment. I love you sooo much.

Chef Dave

Contents

Foreword

Congratulations! You are about to embark upon a culinary journey that is truly inspirational!

The recipes in this book combine wonderful tastes with a 21st century modernity that embraces our desire for greater fitness and longevity. The pages of this book present a captivating array of flavors from around the world that challenge the reader to think beyond any previously held notions of nutrition and healthy eating.

This book shows that you can eat healthy and still enjoy superb cuisine. The scents and sights of these creations are themselves sinful. And any lingering doubts that the power and creativity of a world-class Chef like Dave Fouts will lift your palate to new heights of eating pleasure will vanish when you've tasted the first bites of his salmon nicoise salad for lunch or the fiesta pasta with rib eye steak for dinner.

The medical evidence is overwhelming that our choices define who we become. And in this age of the proliferation of unhealthy temptations on nearly every street corner and grocery isle, I congratulate you on selecting this superb choice of healthy and delicious cuisine for you and your family.

Enjoy! You will not be disappointed.

Kent C. Sasse, MD, MPH, FACS
Medical Director, Western Bariatric Institute
Founder, International Metabolic Institute™
Author, **Outpatient Weight Loss Surgery**
Author, **Doctor's Orders**
Author, **Life Changing Weight Loss**

www.sasseguide.com

Introduction from Chef Dave

When writing "Ditch Your Diet in 30 Days" the goal was to create a monthly meal plan that anybody could follow. The food had to be available without making extra trips to specialty food markets. The menu had to be simple enough to follow, and the recipes had to be quick. In addition there had to be plenty of variety. I believe the number one reason eating healthy does not always work is lack of flavor and texture, and "Ditch Your Diet in 30 Days" breaks through the food flavor barrier.

Hunger while maintaining and losing weight has always been an issue, and I wanted to make sure that not only three balanced meals were eaten, but 3 snacks a day as well, and all of this within a 1200 calorie meal plan. Within this book your taste buds will be excited, and your stomach content.

It's gotta be easy! Nothing could be truer, and within this book you will find easy and time managed recipes to fit into even the busiest schedule. Not only are fresh ingredients used, but convenience foods such as prepackaged fish, chicken, and seafood to help speed up those lunch time needs. It was now important to me to not only create great dishes but to keep them simple.

"I don't have time" is a phrase I have often hear when it comes to eating and taking care of our bodies. So creating recipes that are packed with flavor and fresh ingredients, but kept under 20 minutes prep time can be a challenge. "Ditch Your Diet in 30 Days" is the key to opening your palate and kitchen to fast and exciting recipes.

All recipes have been created and personally tested in my own kitchen and you have my promise that all the recipes have been developed not only for my weight loss surgery friends, but to those who desire healthy eating for weight management.

Cook Smart
Chef Dave Fouts

Before You Begin

Valuable Comments from Chef Dave

Life is complicated. Whether you are a single person with a job to manage or a mother of three racing to the soccer field, juggling it all can be a full time and often overwhelming task. In this age of the proliferation of unhealthy food temptations on nearly every street corner and grocery isle, making poor choices for yourself and your family has been made that much easier. Food marketing is a vast science. Manufacturers and restaurateurs know how to appeal to our overburdened schedules by making highly processed, high fat, high carbohydrate foods seem irresistible. The only way to protect yourself from this bombardment is to be proactive and knowledgeable about what good nutrition really is and where to find it.

If you have found yourself carrying unwanted weight as a result of a diet too rich in these unhealthy foods, don't despair. If you are beginning a weight loss journey as the first step to better health, good for you! This book will be a powerful weapon to add to your arsenal as you move your eating choices to the healthy end of the spectrum.

Let's take a moment to consider some key behaviors that I've learned and science has well proven to work for losing and even more importantly, maintaining weight. If followed, these changes will greatly assist you in achieving your weight loss goals and in establishing the critical groundwork for a healthy life for the long term.

Take ownership of what you eat...

Don't be someone who is looking for an outside force to do the work of creating weight loss or someone who's going to say, "The diet didn't work" as soon as the results aren't there. The downfall behind the idea is that the diet (or pills or shots or hypnosis or any other outside solution or force or magic) is going to do all the work. Of course not. You are.

Don't get caught in this syndrome. Take ownership of your life and your health and your weight. Only you have the power to change and succeed. You have the tools – go for the success.

1) Eat six times a day - Most of us are of the opinion that starving and/or skipping meals is the most obvious and rapid way to drop unwanted pounds. Many of us again, because of busy schedules or bad habits, skip meals on a regular basis, most often breakfast. Strangely enough, you can gain weight by doing that. When you skip meals or eat on an inconsistent schedule, what you actually do is teach your body not to trust you to feed it. Then on the chance that food will be scarce, when you do eat, your body will store the calories for later use rather than burn them off. This slows your metabolism as your body goes into "starvation mode" and can result in weight gain.

By eating six small meals a day and eating them every three hours or so, your metabolism will speed up, your blood sugar will remain stable and your brain will get the message to treat the food as "fuel" and burn off the calories.

Having the appropriate foods on hand for these 6 meals will require active planning. That will mean you need to put taking care of your body and its needs somewhere on that packed calendar every day. If you spend time mapping out your menu for the week and doing some advanced food preparation, you and your family can eat very well and leave the processed foods behind.

2) *Protein, protein, protein!* - There is no question that becoming a smart grocery shopper is necessary for success. This means you need to learn how to read labels and educate yourself about the nutritional value/cost of the foods you eat. 100 calorie packs are all the rage in stores right now. The food companies are preying on the public's general desire for better health. They attempt to convince us that by eating 100 calorie controlled portions, we are making good food choices. Certainly while the caloric level is acceptable for a snack and may facilitate eating less at one sitting, almost all the foods packaged in this manner are largely empty carbohydrates.

Turn your focus to protein instead. This book has terrific recipes that do just that. Eating protein keeps your blood sugar stable so you don't get cravings. When you eat carbohydrates, they set up a vicious cycle of cravings and will cause large fluctuations in your blood sugar levels. That big energy crash and fatigue you experience in the middle of the afternoon is likely due to the amount of carbohydrates you ate at lunch time.

Eating protein is also critical in its support of lean mass maintenance and development. Your dry lean mass (muscle) is the mechanism that burns your calories. Often rapid weight loss can result in the loss of lean mass and in turn, a reduction in the number of calories your body burns. Eating adequate protein, when combined with exercise can maintain and even increase lean mass.

Again, there are many foods available now that tout the protein they contain. Don't be seduced by this marketing angle. Look at the label and see how many calories and carbohydrates the food contains. Adding a few grams of protein does not turn a cookie into a chicken breast! Always look for the choices that have the fewest carbs and the most protein for the calories. It is always best to shop around the perimeter of your grocery store where the fresh meats, vegetables and dairy are and stay out of the center of the store where many of the highly processed foods are lurking. Convenience can often be nutritionally costly.

3) Watch your portions - Whether you are at your goal weight or still working on it, one of the easiest ways to undermine your success is to have "too much of a good thing". If you are making better or good choices you can still get in trouble if you eat too much of it. While vegetables generally have low caloric and carbohydrate count, fruit contains a fair amount of carbs. Take time to learn what an appropriate portion for any given food is 3 oz. of protein (about the size of the palm of your hand), a half cup of starch and a half plate of salad or vegetables are reasonable.

4) Determine your "triggers" - Don't take your new body into your old life. These are situations, places, emotions that cause you to respond by eating. It could be whenever you are stressed, bored, sitting in front of the TV or driving home after work. They are different for everyone. If you don't take the time to get a handle on what yours are, you will be at risk to put weight back on (or not take it off in the first place) because these "life" situations will arise and you will default to the habits you had before. Once you identify them, work in alternatives to food as solutions.

5) Working within your caloric "budget" - If you've "been good" during your active weight loss phase, resuming Friday night pizza with the family or big tubs of popcorn at the movies because it is what you've "always done" will start you down that slippery slope to weight gain again. If you can't be satisfied with a salad while everyone else eats pizza, start a new trend and either eat at a healthier restaurant or introduce a new/different group activity. If you do over-eat or "treat yourself" to something that wasn't the best choice, turn right around and start paying the calories back. Reduce your calories for the next couple of days and/or get more exercise in so that by the end of the week, you're back where you started and within your budget. Using recipes from this book will help you get back on track with tasty, healthy meals.

Congratulations on making the decision to embark on a culinary journey that is truly inspirational! The recipes in this book combine wonderful tastes that embrace our desire for greater fitness and longevity. This book will show you how you can get healthy while enjoying superb cuisine. Use these basic weight loss tips in conjunction with these amazing recipes and find the perfect companions for success.

Cook Smart
Chef Dave Fouts

Healthful Tips from Your Dietitian

Congratulations on your decision to manage your weight and eat more healthfully! There is a lot of information out there to help you down the road to improved health. Some of it can be downright confusing. Chef Dave and I have made every effort to make this journey easier for you. Chef Dave's skills have made the recipes easy and quick to prepare, plus they taste good!

We have developed a menu plan that includes three meals and three snacks a day. This is not grazing. Grazing is the indiscriminate nibbling and picking that goes on all day. Our daily menu has a specified portion of food to be eaten at regular times. Eating fewer than four meals or snacks a day or eating more than six meals or snacks a day increases the risk of obesity. Eating more often reduces hunger. You know what happens when you skip a meal. The next meal is eaten too fast; most likely you eat too much, and usually we don't make the best food choices.

So if you are eating six times a day that means you need to eat breakfast. People who skip breakfast are more likely to become obese than breakfast eaters. Studies have shown that people who ate breakfast ate less at later meals and were less likely to get into trouble with snacking. While running to the coffee shop and picking up a designer drink or a pastry may be easy, it doesn't provide much in the way meeting your nutrient goals but does contribute to significant calories. I know it can be a rush to get out the door in the morning so we have included breakfast items that take less time than sitting in the drive-thru.

How often have you come home from work and said, "What's for dinner?" How often has the answer been, "I don't know. Let's go out." With some forethought and planning you can eat healthy, easy meals at home. The first step to eating more meals at home is to plan a menu. We have done the work for you and given tasty meals that are easy to prepare with foods that come from your regular food store, not the specialty ones. We have even made your grocery list! Check your pantry staples on our list because these food items will come up often in our menu plan. Each week has a shopping list developed from the recipes for that week. You will need to check the snack lists and add your snack items to our shopping list.

You may also notice that our shopping list includes a lot of produce. Your mom was right when she said to eat your fruits and vegetables. Eating more fruits and vegetables is likely to reduce the risk of chronic diseases such as stroke, cardiovascular disease, type 2 diabetes, and certain cancers. Plus they are important for calorie control. Most fruits and vegetables are low in calories but high in fiber that can help you feel fuller longer. They are also chock full of vitamins and minerals. Chef Dave and I have worked together to make the menus meet most recommended dietary guidelines. As long as you follow the menus we have provided you don't need to count calories, grams of protein, carbohydrates or fat or worry about eating too much cholesterol or sodium. The fewer decisions you have to make about what to eat and when to eat it will make it easier for you to stay on a plan. You'll have more time to spend on those things in your life that are more important. Just remember, if you change the serving size or substitute ingredients or side dishes, you will change the nutrition information provided on our meal labels.

We have modified the USDA and FDA Nutrition Facts Label for our meal plans and daily menus. You will see a Facts Label for each meal, each day's menu, and a label for the weekly average of all meals for all days in the week. If you are reading the food labels on packaged foods, our labels will make it a snap for you to determine the nutritional value.

The nutrition information for the daily menus will vary slightly with your snack choices. The nutritional values for the snacks were based on the average amount of each nutrient for all foods listed in the snack list. Choose a wide variety of foods from the snack lists to meet daily nutritional needs. Because our menus are "bariatric friendly", meaning portions and foods have been adjusted for post operative weight loss surgery patients, you may want to choose fruits and vegetables from the snack lists to help you feel fuller. Each recipe and menu have been analyzed with ESHA Research Food Processor SQL software, Version 9.9 (Salem, OR).

Following our menu plans takes the guesswork out of how much and when to eat. They also provide you healthy, easy meals totaling 1200 calories a day to help you meet your weight loss and weight management goals.

Eat Smart
Vicki Bovee, M.S., R.D.

Understanding Label Facts

Example Menu - Day 26

Breakfast

o Guiltless Shrimp and Brie Scrambled Eggs with Whole Wheat English Muffin

Mid Morning Snack

o 100 Calorie Snack

Lunch

o Pork Arroz Con Queso

Mid Afternoon Snack

o 100 Calorie Snack

Dinner

o Pan Seared Tilapia on Linguini with Tomato Cream Sauce

Evening Snack

o 100 Calorie Snack

Nutrition Facts
Daily Menu

Amount Per Serving	
Calories 1200	Calories from Fat 315

Total Fat 35g	
Saturated Fat 13g	
Trans Fat 0g	
Cholesterol 255mg	
Sodium 1925mg	
Total Carbohydrate 123g	
Dietary Fiber 18g	
Sugars 35g	
Protein 98g	

Calories Per Gram:
Fat 9 – Carbohydrate 4 – Protein 4

You don't have to hire your own personal chef or be a gourmet cook to prepare delicious, easy, and healthy meals. You don't need to be a dietitian to figure out if you are eating a nutritionally balanced diet. Chef Dave and I have given you Ditch Your Diet in 30 Days to make it happen. Enjoy!

- Vicki Bovee, M.S., R.D.

Serving

The serving on the label is the amount or daily total for one person.

Calories

The total calories for each meal includes the recommended side dish. The total calories for each day range from 1190 to 1210 calories per day, including snacks.

Total Fat

Eating too much fat may increase your risk for certain chronic diseases. Dietary goals for fat are 20-35% of total calories for the day. If you are eating 1200 calories per day, that equals 27 to 47 grams of fat a day. Our meal plans average 28% of total calories, or 37 grams of fat per day.

Saturated Fat

Too much saturated fat can increase your bad cholesterol levels. Dietary goals for saturated fats are less than 10% of total calories. Our meal plans average 8% of total calories from saturated fats.

Trans Fat

These are the worst of all fats and can raise bad (LDL) cholesterol levels. The less the better...

Cholesterol

A diet high in dietary cholesterol can increase your bad cholesterol levels and increases your risk of developing heart disease. Recommendations are an intake of less than 300mg per day. Our meal plans average 217mg of cholesterol per day.

Sodium

Too much sodium can lead to high blood pressure and other health problems. Most of the sodium in our daily diet comes from processed and prepared foods. We have used low sodium products in many of our recipes. Remember if you substitute a low sodium ingredient such as low sodium chicken broth with regular chicken broth, you will increase your sodium intake above the recommended amounts. The recommended amount of sodium is less than 2300mg per day. Our meal plans average 1960 mg sodium per day.

Total Carbohydrates

Carbohydrates provide energy to all cells in our body. A healthy diet includes carbohydrates from whole grains and fruits and vegetables. We have used whole grain breads, pastas, rice, and tortillas instead of refined white flour products. The minimum recommended daily intake for carbohydrates is 100 grams per day. Our meal plans average 129 grams per day, or 43% of total calories for the day.

Fiber

A diet higher in fiber can help with weight loss, help lower cholesterol, help control blood sugar, and help keep your digestive system regular. Recommendations are 14 grams of fiber per 1000 calories. If you are eating 1200 calories a day, that is 17 grams of fiber a day. Our daily meal plans average 21 grams of fiber a day.

Sugar

Sugar in food comes from the naturally occurring sugar in food like milk products and fruits, or from added sugars. The recommendations are for less than 25% of total calories from added sugars. Our recipes include almost no added sugars. If you are monitoring the amount of sugar you are consuming in a meal, the sugar in our recipes comes from the food itself, not from added sugars, and should not cause problems with dumping syndrome if you have had weight loss surgery.

Protein

Most Americans do not have a problem eating enough protein every day. If you have had weight loss surgery, you may find it difficult to meet the protein requirements set by your surgeon. Our meal plans average 89 grams of protein a day. You can increase this by choosing protein-based snacks from the snack lists. The recommendations are 10-35% of total calories from protein. Our meal plans average 30% of total calories from protein.

Pantry Staples

These foods will be used throughout the 30 day menu plan. We have included a weekly shopping list for recipe specific foods.

Baking Products
almond extract
baking powder
baking soda
brown sugar
granulated sugar
nonfat dry powdered milk
Splenda®
vanilla extract

Condiments
Dijon mustard
ketchup
mayonnaise, light
salsa
Tabasco® sauce
Worcestershire sauce

Cooking Oils
balsamic vinegar
canola oil
cider vinegar
olive oil
red wine vinegar
white vinegar
white wine vinegar

Flours
all-purpose flour
cornstarch

Spices and Seasonings
apple pie spice
bay leaves
black pepper
caraway seeds
cayenne pepper
chili powder
cinnamon
crushed rosemary
curry powder
dried basil
dried dill
dried italian seasoning
dried marjoram
dried oregano
dried sage
dried tarragon
dry mustard
garlic powder
ground coriander
ground cumin
ground thyme
lemon pepper
ground nutmeg
onion powder
paprika
peppercorns
pumpkin pie spice
red pepper flakes
taco seasoning mix
white pepper

Daily Nutritional Average

Nutrition Facts
Weekly Daily Average

Amount Per Serving

Calories 1200 Calories from Fat 335

Total Fat 37g

  Saturated Fat 9.5g

  Trans Fat 0g

Cholesterol 225mg

Sodium 2105mg

Total Carbohydrate 130g

  Dietary Fiber 22g

  Sugars 40g

Protein 87g

Calories Per Gram:
  Fat 9 – Carbohydrate 4 – Protein 4

Week 1 Recipes

Day 1   Classic Egg and Cheese Breakfast Sandwich
Hurry Curry Pork Salad
Chicken Cacciatore

Day 2   Chived Herb Baked Eggs
Open-Face Turkey Avocado Sandwich
Oven-Fried Pecan Catfish

Day 3   Chunky Banana Almond Oatmeal
Crab Papaya Confetti Salad
Home-Style Chicken in Tomato Gravy

Day 4   Scrumptious Salmon Omelet
Shaved Ham and Havarti Salad in Pita Pockets
Layered Chicken and Shrimp Enchilada Casserole

Day 5   Muesli with Yogurt and Raspberries
Santa Fe Turkey Salad
Fiesta Pasta with Rib Eye Steak

Day 6   Asparagus and Ham Roll 'em Ups
Tart Cherry Shrimp Salad Lettuce Wraps
Green and White Meatless Lasagna

Day 7   Yummy Sausage and Cheddar Frittata
Salmon Nicoise Salad
Brunswick Stew

Week 1 Shopping List

Bread Products
bread, whole wheat	5 slices
English muffins, whole wheat	4
pita bread, whole wheat	3 small

Canned Beans
black beans, low sodium	2 cups
kidney beans, low sodium	2 15 ounce cans

Canned Fruits
papaya	1 cup
pineapple chunks, in juice	2 cups

Canned Seafood & Meat
crab meat	1 pound
salmon	16 ounces
shrimp	4-1/4 ounces

Canned Vegetables
corn, whole kernel	1/4 cup
corn, Mexican-style	1 cup
potatoes, unsalted	1 cup
tomatoes, low sodium	5 14.5 ounce cans

Cereals
barley flakes	2 tablespoons
oatmeal, instant plain	1 packet
oats, rolled	2 tablespoons

Dairy Products
cheddar cheese, low-fat, sharp	1-1/2 cups shredded
cheddar cheese, low-fat, shredded	2 cups
cream cheese, light	2 ounces
egg whites	2
eggs	1 large
havarti cheese	2 ounces
margarine, light tub	8 teaspoons
margarine, stick	1 tablespoon
milk, 1%	2 cups
milk, nonfat	1-2/3 cups
Monterey jack cheese, low-fat	3 ounces
mozzarella cheese, part skim	8 ounces
parmesan cheese, fresh grated	4 ounces
ricotta cheese, part skim	15 ounces
sour cream, light	1-3/8 cups
sour cream, nonfat	1/2 cup
yogurt, light vanilla	6 ounces
yogurt, nonfat plain	1/4 cup

Deli Lunchmeat
ham slices, lean	1/2 pound
ham slices, low sodium	4 ounces
turkey breast, low sodium	8 ounces
turkey ham	4 ounces

Dried Fruit
cherries, dried tart	1/4 cup
raisins	2 tablespoons

Flours
Wondra® Quick-mixing flour	1/4 cup

Fresh Seafood & Fish
catfish fillets	1 pound
shrimp, fresh	1 pound

Frozen Foods
egg substitute	3 cups
butternut squash	12 ounces
corn, whole kernel	2 cups
lima beans	2 cups
spinach, chopped	10 ounces

Jams & Jellies
strawberry 100% fruit spread	6 tablespoons

Meat & Poultry
beef, rib eye steak	8 ounces
chicken breasts, boneless skinless	6 pounds
pork tenderloin	1 pound
turkey sausage, fresh	6 ounces
turkey breast, ground	1 pound

Mexican Food Products

tortillas, corn	24
green chilies, canned	1 tablespoon
tortillas, whole wheat	4 small

Nuts & Seeds

almonds, slivered	3 tablespoons
pecans	2 ounces
walnuts	2 teaspoons

Pasta

pasta, whole wheat, lasagna	9 pieces
pasta, whole wheat, penne	3 cups
pasta, whole wheat	1/2 cup

Pickles & Olives

black olives, sliced	5 ounces

Produce

apple	1 medium
asparagus	18 spears
avocados	1 medium
bananas	2 medium
basil leaves, fresh	1 tablespoon
Bibb lettuce	1 cup
broccoli flowerets	1-1/2 pounds
butterhead lettuce	2 cups
cantaloupe	1 large
carrot	1 medium
carrots, baby	4 cups
celery	1 stalk
cherry tomatoes	1/2 cup
chives, fresh	2 teaspoons
cucumbers	1/2 medium
garlic	7 cloves
grapes	20
green beans	1-1/4 pounds
leaf lettuce	3 cups
lemon juice, fresh	2 lemons
lime juice	1 tablespoon
mixed salad greens	2 cups
onion, red	1 medium
onions, green	5
onions, yellow	7 medium
orange	1/2 medium
oregano, fresh	1 teaspoon
parsley, fresh	1 bunch
peaches	4 medium
peppers, green bell	5 medium
pepper, red bell	1 small
plums	6
radishes	6 small
raspberries	1/2 cup
romaine lettuce	3 cups
tomato	3 small
tomatoes, plum	3 large
zucchini	2 medium

Snack Foods

oyster crackers	2 cups
whole wheat crackers, reduced fat	24

Soups

chicken broth, low sodium	1 cup

Cooking Spirits

white wine	1/2 cup

Tomato Sauces

tomato paste	6 ounces
tomato paste, low sodium	8 ounces
tomato puree	16 ounces
tomato puree, unsalted	16 ounces

Daily Menu

Breakfast
- o Classic Egg and Cheese Breakfast Sandwich with Fresh Orange

Mid Morning Snack
- o 100 Calorie Snack

Lunch
- o Hurry Curry Pork Salad with Reduced Fat Whole Wheat Crackers

Mid Afternoon Snack
- o 100 Calorie Snack

Dinner
- o Chicken Cacciatore with Green Beans and Penne Pasta

Evening Snack
- o 75 Calorie Snack

Nutrition Facts
Daily Menu
Amount Per Serving
Calories 1200 Calories from Fat 305
Total Fat 34g
Saturated Fat 7g
Trans Fat 0g
Cholesterol 389mg
Sodium 2005mg
Total Carbohydrate 133g
Dietary Fiber 23g
Sugars 47g
Protein 92g
Calories Per Gram: Fat 9 – Carbohydrate 4 – Protein 4

Breakfast

Classic Egg and Cheese Breakfast Sandwich
with Fresh Orange

Serves 1

1	**whole wheat English muffin, toasted**
1 large	**egg**
1 tablespoon	**low-fat cheddar cheese, shredded**
1 teaspoon	**low-fat margarine**
1 medium	**orange, half**

Directions

1. Add margarine to small sauté pan and cook over medium heat until margarine is melted.

2. Add egg and cheese to melted margarine and stir with plastic spatula until egg is cooked and cheese is melted (approximately 3-4 minutes).

3. Serve cooked egg and cheese over toasted English muffin.

Serve with 1/2 fresh orange.

Nutrition Facts

Servings Per Meal: 1

Amount Per Serving

Calories 280   Calories from Fat 100

Total Fat 11g	
Saturated Fat 2.5g	
Trans Fat 0g	
Cholesterol 215mg	
Sodium 400mg	
Total Carbohydrate 34g	
Dietary Fiber 6g	
Sugars 13g	
Protein 15g	

Calories Per Gram:
Fat 9 – Carbohydrate 4 – Protein 4

6

Lunch

Hurry Curry Pork Salad
with Reduced Fat Whole Wheat Crackers

Serves 6

1 pound	lean pork tenderloin, cooked and cut into thin strips
1-1/2 medium	apple, peeled and chopped
1	banana, sliced
2 tablespoons	raisins, plumped*
1/3 cup	light mayonnaise
2 tablespoons	chutney, chopped
1/2 teaspoon	curry powder
24	reduced fat whole wheat crackers

Nutrition Facts

Servings Per Meal: 6

Amount Per Serving

Calories 290   Calories from Fat 90

Total Fat 11g

Saturated Fat 1.5g

Trans Fat 0g

Cholesterol 65mg

Sodium 240mg

Total Carbohydrate 26g

Dietary Fiber 3g

Sugars 7g

Protein 23g

Calories Per Gram:
Fat 9 – Carbohydrate 4 – Protein 4

Directions

1. In large bowl, mix pork, apple, banana, and raisins.

2. Mix mayonnaise, chutney, and curry powder in small bowl and pour over salad, stirring lightly to coat.

To serve, divide mixture into 6 equal portions and serve each with 4 whole wheat crackers.

*Note: To plump raisins, place them in a heat resistant bowl and cover with one cup boiling water for five minutes and then drain liquid. Raisins are now plumped.

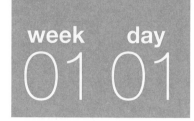

Dinner
Chicken Cacciatore
with Green Beans and Whole Wheat Penne

Serves 8

2 pounds	boneless skinless chicken breasts
3 tablespoons	all-purpose flour
1/8 teaspoon	black pepper
1 teaspoon	salt
1 tablespoon	olive oil
1 medium	onion, sliced
2 cloves	garlic, minced
2 tablespoons	fresh parsley, minced
1/ 2 teaspoon	oregano
1/2 cup	carrots, chopped
1/2 cup	celery, chopped
16 ounces	unsalted canned tomatoes, chopped
1/2 cup	white wine
6 ounces	tomato paste
1 pound	green beans, cooked
3 cups	whole wheat pasta, cooked

Nutrition Facts

Nutrition Facts

Servings Per Meal: 8

Amount Per Serving

Calories 280   Calories from Fat 30

Total Fat 3.5g

   Saturated Fat 0.5g

   Trans Fat 0g

Cholesterol 65mg

Sodium 580mg

Total Carbohydrate 30g

   Dietary Fiber 6g

   Sugars 7g

Protein 32g

Calories Per Gram:
Fat 9 – Carbohydrate 4 – Protein 4

Directions

1. Mix together flour, salt, and pepper. Coat chicken with mixture; set aside.

2. Add olive oil to medium size sauce pan and heat on very low temperature.

3. Add onions to pan and sauté until light brown.

4. Add chicken and sauté until browned.

5. Stir in garlic, parsley, oregano, carrots, celery, tomatoes, white wine and tomato paste.

6. Bring to a simmer; cook covered for 20 minutes.

To serve, divide chicken cacciatore into 8 equal portions and serve each over pasta and top with steamed green beans.

Daily Menu

Breakfast
o Chived Herb Baked Eggs with Cantaloupe

Mid Morning Snack
o 100 Calorie Snack

Lunch
o Open-Face Turkey Avocado Sandwich with Grapes

Mid Afternoon Snack
o 100 Calorie Snack

Dinner
o Oven-Fried Pecan Catfish with Butternut Squash

Evening Snack
o 75 Calorie Snack

Nutrition Facts	
Daily Menu	
Amount Per Serving	
Calories 1200	Calories from Fat 440
Total Fat 49g	
Saturated Fat 9g	
Trans Fat 0g	
Cholesterol 145mg	
Sodium 2000mg	
Total Carbohydrate 112g	
Dietary Fiber 20g	
Sugars 40g	
Protein 78g	

Calories Per Gram:
Fat 9 – Carbohydrate 4 – Protein 4

Breakfast
Chived Herb Baked Eggs
with Cantaloupe

Serves 6

1/4 pound	turkey ham, finely chopped
2 cups	egg substitute
2 teaspoons	Dijon mustard
1/2 cup	fat-free sour cream
2 teaspoons	fresh chives, chopped
2 teaspoons	fresh parsley, chopped
3/4 cup	low-fat cheddar cheese, shredded
1 large	cantaloupe, peeled and cubed

Directions

1. Preheat oven to 375° F.

2. Spray 8 x 8 inch non-stick baking pan with vegetable coating; add turkey ham.

3. Whisk together egg substitute, mustard, and sour cream; add to pan.

4. Stir in herbs and top with shredded cheese.

5. Bake 25-30 minutes until golden and set.

To serve, divide eggs into 6 equal portions and serve each with 1 cup cubed cantaloupe.

Nutrition Facts
Servings Per Meal: 6

Amount Per Serving

Calories 190   Calories from Fat 45

Total Fat 5g

   Saturated Fat 1.5g

   Trans Fat 0g

Cholesterol 25mg

Sodium 520mg

Total Carbohydrate 18g

   Dietary Fiber 2g

   Sugars 14g

Protein 20g

Calories Per Gram:
   Fat 9 – Carbohydrate 4 – Protein 4

Lunch
Open-Face Turkey Avocado Sandwich
with Grapes

Serves 1

1 slice	whole wheat bread
1-1/2 teaspoons	light mayonnaise
1/2 medium	avocado, peeled and sliced
2 ounces	low sodium deli turkey
2 slices	tomatoes
20	grapes

Directions

1. Spread mayo over bread and layer with turkey, tomatoes, and avocado.

2. Cut in half.

Serve with grapes.

Nutrition Facts

Servings Per Meal: *1*

Amount Per Serving

Calories 380 Calories from Fat 170

Total Fat 18g

Saturated Fat 2g

Trans Fat 0g

Cholesterol 30mg

Sodium 500mg

Total Carbohydrate 43g

Dietary Fiber 10g

Sugars 19g

Protein 19g

Calories Per Gram:
Fat 9 – Carbohydrate 4 – Protein 4

Dinner
Oven-Fried Pecan Catfish
with Butternut Squash

Serves 4

3 tablespoons	Dijon mustard
1/3 cup	nonfat milk
2 ounces	pecans, chopped fine
1 pound	catfish filet, divided into 4 equal portions
12 ounces	frozen butternut squash
1/2 teaspoon	cinnamon

Directions

1. Preheat oven to 450° F.

2. Mix Dijon mustard and milk in a shallow bowl.

3. Spread pecans onto parchment paper or foil.

4. Coat each catfish filet with Dijon mixture, and then roll into ground pecans, shaking off excess.

5. Place prepared fish onto lightly oiled baking sheet.

6. Bake until catfish flakes easily when tested with a fork, approximately 10-12 minutes.

7. Heat butternut squash according to package directions and sprinkle with cinnamon.

Serve each piece of fish with 1/4 cup butternut squash.

Nutrition Facts

Servings Per Meal: 4

Amount Per Serving

Calories 320   Calories from Fat 170

Total Fat 19g

Saturated Fat 3g

Trans Fat 0g

Cholesterol 55mg

Sodium 340mg

Total Carbohydrate 17g

Dietary Fiber 2g

Sugars 4g

Protein 21g

Calories Per Gram:
Fat 9 – Carbohydrate 4 – Protein 4

Daily Menu

Breakfast

o Chunky Banana Almond Oatmeal

Mid Morning Snack

o 100 Calorie Snack

Lunch

o Crab Papaya Confetti Salad

Mid Afternoon Snack

o 100 Calorie Snack

Dinner

o Home-Style Chicken in Tomato Gravy with Broccoli

Evening Snack

o 75 Calorie Snack

Nutrition Facts
Daily Menu

Amount Per Serving

Calories 1200 Calories from Fat 235

Total Fat 26g

Saturated Fat 4.5g

Trans Fat 0g

Cholesterol 195mg

Sodium 2150mg

Total Carbohydrate 152g

Dietary Fiber 25g

Sugars 45g

Protein 89g

Calories Per Gram:
Fat 9 – Carbohydrate 4 – Protein 4

Breakfast
Chunky Banana Almond Oatmeal

Serves 1

1 packet	**plain instant oatmeal**
1/2 cup	**nonfat milk**
1 medium	**banana, chopped**
1/4 teaspoon	**almond extract**
2 packets	**Splenda®**

Directions

1. Combine oatmeal, nonfat milk, banana, almond extract, and Splenda®.

2. Mix well; cover with plastic wrap.

3. Microwave for 2 minutes 30 seconds, or until oatmeal begins to bubble.

4. Stir and serve.

Nutrition Facts
Servings Per Meal: 1

Amount Per Serving

Calories 340   Calories from Fat 40

Total Fat 4.5g

Saturated Fat 0.5g

Trans Fat 0g

Cholesterol 0mg

Sodium 250mg

Total Carbohydrate 65g

Dietary Fiber 7g

Sugars 21g

Protein 11g

Calories Per Gram:
Fat 9 – Carbohydrate 4 – Protein 4

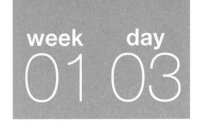

Lunch
Crab Papaya Confetti Salad

Serves 4

Dressing:

2 tablespoons	olive oil
1/2 teaspoon	garlic powder
2 teaspoons	Dijon mustard
1/2 teaspoon	black pepper
1 tablespoon	lime juice
2 tablespoons	fresh parsley, chopped fine

Directions

1. Combine dressing ingredients in a bowl. Refrigerate and set aside.

Salad:

1 pound	crab meat, canned or in pouch
2 cups	mixed salad greens
1 cup	canned low-sodium black beans, rinsed and drained
1/4 cup	canned corn, drained
1 cup	canned papaya, chopped

Directions

1. In large bowl add crab meat, salad greens, black beans, corn kernels, and papaya.

2. Pour dressing over salad; mix and serve.

Nutrition Facts

Servings Per Meal: 4

Amount Per Serving

Calories 260   Calories from Fat 70

Total Fat 9g

Saturated Fat 1g

Trans Fat 0g

Cholesterol 85mg

Sodium 630mg

Total Carbohydrate 20g

Dietary Fiber 4g

Sugars 8g

Protein 29g

Calories Per Gram:
Fat 9 – Carbohydrate 4 – Protein 4

Dinner
Home-Style Chicken in Tomato Gravy
with Broccoli

Serves 4

1 pound	**boneless skinless chicken breasts, divided into 4 equal portions**
1/4 cup	**Wondra® Quick-mixing flour**
1/2 teaspoon	**black pepper**
1 tablespoon	**canola oil**
1 large	**onion, finely chopped**
2 large	**green peppers, chopped**
1 clove	**garlic, minced**
1/4 teaspoon	**white pepper**
1-1/2 teaspoons	**curry powder**
16 ounces	**tomato puree**
1 teaspoon	**parsley, chopped**
1/4 teaspoon	**ground thyme**
2 cups	**broccoli florets, steamed**

Nutrition Facts

Servings Per Meal: 4

Amount Per Serving

Calories 300   Calories from Fat 50

Total Fat 6g

   Saturated Fat 1g

   Trans Fat 0g

Cholesterol 65mg

Sodium 540mg

Total Carbohydrate 33g

   Dietary Fiber 8g

   Sugars 12g

Protein 32g

Calories Per Gram:
   Fat 9 – Carbohydrate 4 – Protein 4

Directions

1. Mix together flour and pepper in large plastic bag.
2. Add chicken, one piece at a time, shaking to coat.
3. Heat oil in large sauté pan.
4. Over medium heat, sauté chicken until brown on both sides and cooked thoroughly.
5. Remove chicken from pan and keep warm.
6. In same sauté pan, stir fry onions, green pepper, and garlic for approximately 5 minutes, until onion is golden brown.
7. Add white pepper, curry powder, tomato puree, chopped parsley, thyme, and chicken.
8. Simmer chicken in tomato gravy for approximately 10 minutes, or until chicken is done.

To serve, divide into 4 equal portions and serve each with 1/2 cup steamed broccoli florets.

Daily Menu

Breakfast

o Scrumptious Salmon Omelet with Whole Wheat Toast

Mid Morning Snack

o 125 Calorie Snack

Lunch

o Shaved Ham and Havarti Salad in Pita Pockets
   with Pineapple

Mid Afternoon Snack

o 75 Calorie Snack

Dinner

o Layered Chicken and Shrimp Enchilada Casserole

Evening Snack

o 75 Calorie Snack

Nutrition Facts
Daily Menu

Amount Per Serving

Calories 1200 Calories from Fat 370

Total Fat 41g	
Saturated Fat 12g	
Trans Fat 0g	
Cholesterol 215mg	
Sodium 2350mg	
Total Carbohydrate 117g	
Dietary Fiber 20g	
Sugars 29g	
Protein 92g	

Calories Per Gram:
   Fat 9 – Carbohydrate 4 – Protein 4

Breakfast
Scrumptious Salmon Omelet
with Whole Wheat Toast

Serves 4

7-1/2 ounces	canned salmon
1 cup	egg substitute
4 tablespoons	light sour cream
1/4 teaspoon	dried tarragon
1 dash	black pepper
1 tablespoon	stick margarine
4 slices	whole wheat bread, toasted
4 teaspoons	light tub margarine

Directions

1. Drain salmon and flake.

2. Beat together egg substitute, sour cream, and tarragon; season lightly with pepper.

3. Melt stick margarine in non-stick pan; add egg mixture and cook over moderate heat until base is set.

4. Arrange salmon over top of omelet and place pan under pre-heated broiler until omelet is set.

5. Loosen omelet onto a serving plate and carefully fold in half.

To serve, divide omelet into 4 equal portions and serve with 1 slice whole wheat toast coated with one teaspoon light margarine.

Nutrition Facts
Servings Per Meal: 4

Amount Per Serving

Calories 270   Calories from Fat 120

Total Fat 13g

Saturated Fat 2g

Trans Fat 0g

Cholesterol 45mg

Sodium 570mg

Total Carbohydrate 15g

Dietary Fiber 2g

Sugars 3g

Protein 25g

Calories Per Gram:
Fat 9 – Carbohydrate 4 – Protein 4

Lunch
Shaved Ham, Turkey, and Havarti Salad in Pita Pockets
with Pineapple

Serves 4

4 ounces	reduced sodium lean ham*, shaved
6 ounces	low sodium turkey breast*, shaved
2 ounces	havarti cheese, shredded
3 cups	romaine lettuce, torn
2 small	tomatoes, diced
1/2 medium	cucumber, peeled and sliced
1 small	green bell pepper, sliced
1 small	onion, cut into rings
6 small	radishes, thinly sliced
1/2 cup	fresh parsley, chopped
1 clove	garlic, crushed

Dressing:

2 tablespoons	olive oil
2 tablespoons	lemon juice
1 teaspoon	dried Italian seasoning
4 small	whole wheat pita pocket
2 cups	canned pineapple chunks in own juice, drained

Nutrition Facts

Nutrition Facts

Servings Per Meal: 4

Amount Per Serving

Calories 350   Calories from Fat 120

Total Fat 14g

Saturated Fat 5g

Trans Fat 0g

Cholesterol 45mg

Sodium 640mg

Total Carbohydrate 38g

Dietary Fiber 6g

Sugars 17g

Protein 22g

Calories Per Gram:
Fat 9 – Carbohydrate 4 – Protein 4

Directions

1. Combine ham, turkey, cheese, lettuce, tomatoes, cucumber, bell pepper, onion, radishes, parsley, and garlic in a large salad bowl.

2. For dressing, whisk together in small bowl the olive oil, lemon juice, and Italian seasoning.

3. Stuff each small pita with salad mixture and drizzle with dressing.

Serve each portion with 1/2 cup pineapple.

*Note: You may substitute shrimp, tuna, or crab for this recipe.

Dinner
Layered Chicken and Shrimp Enchilada Casserole

Serves 12

1 tablespoon	canola oil
1 pound	shrimp, peeled and deveined
1 pound	boneless skinless chicken breast, cut into half-inch cubes
1 large	onion, chopped
2 cloves	garlic, minced
28 ounces	canned tomatoes, diced
15 ounces	unsalted canned pureed tomatoes
2 tablespoons	chili powder
2 teaspoons	cumin
1 cup	low-sodium canned black beans, drained
1/4 cup	black olives, sliced
2 teaspoons	cilantro
2 cups	low-fat cheddar cheese, shredded
24	corn tortillas
3/4 cup	light sour cream
3/4 cup	salsa

Nutrition Facts
Servings Per Meal: 12

Amount Per Serving

Calories 310   Calories from Fat 60

Total Fat 7g

Saturated Fat 2.5g

Trans Fat 0g

Cholesterol 90mg

Sodium 460mg

Total Carbohydrate 36g

Dietary Fiber 6g

Sugars 5g

Protein 27g

Calories Per Gram:
Fat 9 – Carbohydrate 4 – Protein 4

Directions
1. Preheat oven to 350° F.
2. Heat oil in large skillet; and add shrimp, chicken, onions, and garlic.
3. Brown and drain oil when done.
4. Add diced tomatoes, pureed tomatoes, chili powder, cumin, and black beans.
5. Bring mixture to a boil; cover and simmer 20 minutes.
6. Add olives and cilantro.
7. Line a 9 x 13 inch baking pan with 8 corn tortillas.
8. First, layer one-third of meat mixture over tortillas, then layer with one-third of the cheese. Repeat with remaining ingredients, reserving last one-third of cheese.
9. Bake UNCOVERED for 30 minutes.
10. Sprinkle with remaining cheese and let sit for approximately 15 minutes before serving.
11. Serve with salsa and sour cream.

Daily Menu

Breakfast
o Muesli with Yogurt and Raspberries

Mid Morning Snack
o 125 Calorie Snack

Lunch
o Santa Fe Turkey Salad

Mid Afternoon Snack
o 100 Calorie Snack

Dinner
o Fiesta Pasta with Rib Eye Steak

Evening Snack
o 75 Calorie Snack

Nutrition Facts
Daily Menu

Amount Per Serving

Calories 1200 Calories from Fat 350

Total Fat 39g

Saturated Fat 13g

Trans Fat 0g

Cholesterol 190mg

Sodium 1690mg

Total Carbohydrate 131g

Dietary Fiber 20g

Sugars 27g

Protein 81g

Calories Per Gram:
Fat 9 – Carbohydrate 4 – Protein 4

Breakfast
Muesli with Yogurt and Raspberries

Serves 1

2 tablespoons	**rolled oats**
2 tablespoons	**barley flakes**
2 teaspoons	**walnuts, chopped**
1/2 cup	**raspberries, chopped**
6 ounces	**light vanilla yogurt**

Directions

1. Mix all ingredients into a large bowl and serve.

Nutrition Facts
Servings Per Meal: 1

Amount Per Serving

Calories 230   Calories from Fat 35

Total Fat 4g

Saturated Fat 0g

Trans Fat 0g

Cholesterol 5mg

Sodium 100mg

Total Carbohydrate 41g

Dietary Fiber 3g

Sugars 12g

Protein 10g

Calories Per Gram:
Fat 9 – Carbohydrate 4 – Protein 4

Lunch
Santa Fe Turkey Salad

Serves 6

1/2 teaspoon	canola oil
1 pound	lean ground turkey*
1 medium	green bell pepper, sliced thin
1 medium	onion, sliced
1/2 cup	salsa (from a jar)
8 ounces	unsalted tomato sauce
15 ounces	low-sodium kidney beans, canned, drained, and rinsed
1 cup	Mexican-style corn, canned, and drained
3 cups	leaf lettuce, shredded
3 ounces	sharp cheddar cheese, grated
6 tablespoons	light sour cream

Nutrition Facts

Nutrition Facts
Servings Per Meal: 6

Amount Per Serving

Calories 330   Calories from Fat 120

Total Fat 14g

Saturated Fat 6g

Trans Fat 0g

Cholesterol 80mg

Sodium 520mg

Total Carbohydrate 28g

Dietary Fiber 6g

Sugars 8g

Protein 23g

Calories Per Gram:
Fat 9 – Carbohydrate 4 – Protein 4

Directions

1. In large skillet, heat oil over medium-high heat.

2. Add turkey, green peppers, and onions.

3. Cook for approximately eight minutes, until turkey is cooked.

4. Add salsa, beans, tomato sauce, and corn to mixture; cook until well-heated throughout.

5. Place 1/2 cup lettuce on each of six medium plates; top with warm mixture.

6. Sprinkle 2 teaspoons of cheese evenly on top of each serving and garnish with sour cream.

*Note: You may substitute shrimp, tuna, or crab for this recipe.

Dinner
Fiesta Pasta with Rib Eye Steak

Serves 4

1/2 cup	whole wheat pasta, uncooked
1 tablespoon	canola oil
3/4 cup	onion, chopped
1/2 cup	red bell pepper, chopped
3 large	plum tomatoes, chopped
1/2 cup	red kidney beans, canned, drained, and rinsed
1/4 cup	water
1 tablespoon	green chilies, canned, chopped, and drained
2 teaspoons	taco seasoning mix
1/4 teaspoon	cumin
1/2 teaspoon	garlic powder
1/2 teaspoon	chili powder
1/2 teaspoon	black pepper
3 ounces	low-fat Monterey jack cheese, shredded
8 ounces	beef rib eye, cooked and sliced thin

Nutrition Facts

Nutrition Facts

Servings Per Meal: 4

Amount Per Serving

Calories 310   Calories from Fat 120

Total Fat 14g

Saturated Fat 5g

Trans Fat 0g

Cholesterol 65mg

Sodium 340mg

Total Carbohydrate 22g

Dietary Fiber 4g

Sugars 4g

Protein 26g

Calories Per Gram:
Fat 9 – Carbohydrate 4 – Protein 4

Directions

1. Cook pasta according to package directions; drain.
2. Heat oil in large saucepan over medium heat; add onion and red pepper.
3. Cook five minutes, stirring occasionally or until tender.
4. Add remaining ingredients except cheese and steak; sauté for five minutes over medium high heat.
5. Reduce heat, and then cook uncovered, stirring occasionally for 15 minutes.
6. In another pan, pound rib-eye steak down to 1/4 inch thick and lightly season with salt and pepper to taste.
7. Sauté steak over medium high heat.
8. Cook steak for 2 minutes then turn and cook an additional 2 minutes.
9. Remove from heat and slice thin.
10. Toss cooked pasta with half of the sauce; then spoon remaining sauce over top.
11. Sprinkle with cheese and top with warm rib eye steak.

Daily Menu

Breakfast

o Asparagus and Ham Roll 'em Ups with Fresh Plums

Mid Morning Snack

o 150 Calorie Snack

Lunch

o Tart Cherry Shrimp Salad Lettuce Wraps

Mid Afternoon Snack

o 150 Calorie Snack

Dinner

o Green and White Meatless Lasagna with Steamed Baby Carrots

Evening Snack

o 100 Calorie Snack

Nutrition Facts	
Daily Menu	
Amount Per Serving	
Calories 1200	Calories from Fat 340
Total Fat 38g	
Saturated Fat 12g	
Trans Fat 0g	
Cholesterol 235mg	
Sodium 2345mg	
Total Carbohydrate 131g	
Dietary Fiber 24g	
Sugars 46g	
Protein 84g	

Calories Per Gram:
Fat 9 – Carbohydrate 4 – Protein 4

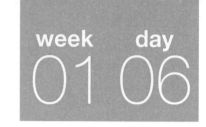

Breakfast
Asparagus and Ham Roll 'em Ups
with Fresh Plums

Serves 6

18	asparagus spears, peeled
1 tablespoon	margarine
1 tablespoon	flour
1/2 teaspoon	dry mustard
1/2 cup	nonfat milk
3/4 cup	low-fat cheddar cheese, grated
6 slices	lean ham, sliced thin
3 tablespoons	almonds, slivered
6 large	plums, seeded and sliced

Directions

1. Preheat oven to 350° F.

2. In nonstick pan, sauté asparagus just until tender (You may use nonstick spray to coat pan first).

3. Melt margarine in heavy saucepan; stir in flour and mustard.

4. Gradually stir in skim milk and cook, stirring constantly until thickened.

5. Add cheese and continue stirring until cheese is melted.

3. Divide asparagus into six portions of three each.

7. Roll each portion of asparagus spears into a slice of ham, in a jelly-roll fashion.

9. Arrange roll-ups in a baking dish with seam sides down.

10. Cover with sauce; bake approximately twenty minutes, until sauce is bubbly, and garnish with almonds.

To serve, divide into 6 portions and serve each with 1 plum.

Nutrition Facts	
Nutrition Facts	
Servings Per Meal: 6	
Amount Per Serving	
Calories 140	Calories from Fat 45
Total Fat 5g	
Saturated Fat 1g	
Trans Fat 0g	
Cholesterol 15mg	
Sodium 420mg	
Total Carbohydrate 13g	
Dietary Fiber 3g	
Sugars 10g	
Protein 11g	
Calories Per Gram:	
Fat 9 – Carbohydrate 4 – Protein 4	

Lunch
Tart Cherry Shrimp Salad Lettuce Wraps

Serves 4

8 ounces	canned shrimp, drained
1/4 cup	dried tart cherries, plumped*
1/2 cup	cherry tomatoes, cut in half
3	green onions, chopped
2 tablespoons	light mayonnaise
2 tablespoons	fat-free plain yogurt
1 tablespoon	fresh lemon juice
1/2 teaspoon	fresh oregano, chopped
1 dash	black pepper
1 cup	Bibb lettuce, chopped
4	whole wheat tortillas

Nutrition Facts
Servings Per Meal: 4

Amount Per Serving

Calories 270   Calories from Fat 60

Total Fat 7g

Saturated Fat 0g

Trans Fat 0g

Cholesterol 120mg

Sodium 410mg

Total Carbohydrate 32g

Dietary Fiber 5g

Sugars 6g

Protein 19g

Calories Per Gram:
Fat 9 – Carbohydrate 4 – Protein 4

Directions

1. In a large bowl, combine shrimp, cherries, tomatoes, and green onions; mix well.

2. Combine mayonnaise, yogurt, lemon juice, oregano, and pepper in a small bowl and pour over shrimp mixture.

3. Mix together gently; refrigerate covered for one to two hours.

4. Place one-quarter of the filling into center of whole wheat tortilla and top with 1/4 cup chopped lettuce.

5. Roll-up and serve.

*Note: To plump cherries place in hot water for 5 minutes; drain and use.

Dinner
Green and White Meatless Lasagna
with Steamed Baby Carrots
Serves 8

9 pieces	whole wheat lasagna noodles, uncooked
1/2 cup	onion, chopped
2 tablespoons	margarine
2 tablespoons	cornstarch
1 tablespoon	parsley
1 teaspoon	dried basil
1/4 teaspoon	garlic powder
1/8 teaspoon	nutmeg
2 cups	1% milk
10 ounces	frozen chopped spinach, thawed and drained
2 1/4 ounces	sliced black olives, drained
8 ounces	part skim milk mozzarella cheese, shredded
1/2 cup	freshly grated parmesan cheese
15 ounces	part skim ricotta cheese
2 large	egg whites, beaten
4 cups	baby carrots, steamed

Nutrition Facts

Servings Per Meal: 8

Amount Per Serving

Calories 390   Calories from Fat 140

Total Fat 16g

Saturated Fat 8g

Trans Fat 0g

Cholesterol 40mg

Sodium 560mg

Total Carbohydrate 37g

Dietary Fiber 8g

Sugars 8g

Protein 24g

Calories Per Gram:
Fat 9 – Carbohydrate 4 – Protein 4

Directions

1. Preheat oven to 350° F.
2. Cook lasagna noodles according to package directions; drain and rinse in cold water; drain well.
3. In a medium saucepan, cook onion in margarine until tender.
4. Stir in cornstarch, parsley, basil, garlic powder, and nutmeg.
5. Add milk all at once and cook stirring constantly until thickened and bubbly.
6. Stir in spinach and olives; add mozzarella and half of the parmesan cheese; mix well.
7. In a medium bowl, stir together ricotta cheese and egg whites.
8. Arrange three of the lasagna pieces onto bottom of a greased 9 x 13 inch baking pan.
9. Top with half of the spinach mixture and half the ricotta mixture; repeat layers.
10. Top with remaining parmesan cheese and bake for 40 minutes or until mixture is bubbly.
11. Let stand 10 minutes.

To serve, divide into 8 equal portions and serve each with 1/2 cup of steamed baby carrots.

Breakfast

o Yummy Sausage and Cheddar Frittata with Whole Wheat English Muffin

Mid Morning Snack

o 100 Calorie Snack

Lunch

o Salmon Nicoise Salad with Fresh Peach

Mid Afternoon Snack

o 150 Calorie Snack

Dinner

o Brunswick Stew with Oyster Crackers

Evening Snack

o 100 Calorie Snack

Nutrition Facts	
Daily Menu	
Amount Per Serving	
Calories 1200	Calories from Fat 290
Total Fat 32g	
Saturated Fat 8g	
Trans Fat 0g	
Cholesterol 190mg	
Sodium 2185mg	
Total Carbohydrate 134g	
Dietary Fiber 22g	
Sugars 46g	
Protein 94g	

Calories Per Gram:
Fat 9 – Carbohydrate 4 – Protein 4

Breakfast
Yummy Sausage and Cheddar Frittata
with Whole Wheat English Muffin

Serves 6

6 ounces	**fresh turkey sausage, sliced**
3 cups	**unpeeled zucchini, shredded**
2	**green onions, chopped**
1 tablespoon	**fresh basil, minced**
1 teaspoon	**Italian seasoning**
1 cup	**egg substitute**
1/3 cup	**nonfat milk**
2 ounces	**light cream cheese, diced into 1/2" cubes**
1/4 cup	**sharp cheddar cheese, shredded**
3	**whole wheat English muffins**
6 tablespoons	**strawberry fruit spread**

Directions

1. Preheat oven to 325° F.

2. Brown sausage and drain well; spread over bottom of greased 8" pie pan or quiche pan.

3. Layer zucchini over sausage; sprinkle green onions and seasonings over top.

4. Whisk egg substitute with milk; pour over zucchini and sausage.

5. Sprinkle with cream cheese cubes; top with cheddar cheese.

6. Bake for 45 minutes until top is lightly golden or knife inserted in center comes out clean.

To serve, divide frittata into 6 equal portions and serve each portion with 1/2 toasted English muffin and 1 tablespoon strawberry spread.

Nutrition Facts
Servings Per Meal: 6

Amount Per Serving

Calories 240   Calories from Fat 70

Total Fat 8g

Saturated Fat 3g

Trans Fat 0g

Cholesterol 30mg

Sodium 520mg

Total Carbohydrate 27g

Dietary Fiber 3g

Sugars 13g

Protein 16g

Calories Per Gram:
Fat 9 – Carbohydrate 4 – Protein 4

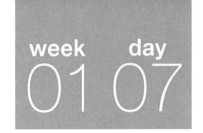

Lunch
Salmon Nicoise Salad
with Fresh Peach

Serves 4

2 cups	butter lettuce
1 cup	green beans, cooked and cooled
1 large	tomato, sliced into wedges
1 small	red bell pepper, cored and sliced
1/2 cup	red onion, thinly sliced
1 cup	unsalted canned potatoes, drained, and chopped
7 1/2 ounces	canned salmon, drained

Classic Vinaigrette:

1 tablespoon	olive oil
1 tablespoon	white wine vinegar
1/4 teaspoon	dry mustard
1 clove	garlic, minced
4 medium	fresh peaches, peeled

Nutrition Facts
Servings Per Meal: 4

Amount Per Serving

Calories 240   Calories from Fat 70

Total Fat 8g

Saturated Fat 1.5g

Trans Fat 0g

Cholesterol 50mg

Sodium 330mg

Total Carbohydrate 24g

Dietary Fiber 6g

Sugars 4g

Protein 22g

Calories Per Gram:
Fat 9 – Carbohydrate 4 – Protein 4

Directions

1. Wash and dry lettuce; arrange leaves on a large serving platter.

2. Toss together beans, tomato wedges, red peppers, red onion slices, and potatoes; arrange onto lettuce leaves.

3. Drain and flake salmon; arrange over bean mixture.

4. To make classic vinaigrette: Whisk together all ingredients until thoroughly combined.

5. Drizzle with classic vinaigrette dressing just before serving.

Serve each portion with a fresh peeled peach.

Dinner
Brunswick Stew
with Oyster Crackers

Serves 8

2 tablespoons	canola oil
2 pounds	boneless skinless chicken breasts
1 teaspoon	paprika
2 medium	onions, sliced
1 medium	green bell pepper, sliced
3 cups	low sodium chicken broth
2 cups	canned tomatoes, not drained
2 tablespoons	fresh parsley, chopped
1/2 teaspoon	Tabasco® sauce
1 tablespoon	Worcestershire sauce
2 cups	whole kernel corn, frozen
2 cups	lima beans, frozen
2 cups	oyster crackers

Directions

1. Heat oil in a deep kettle.

2. Sprinkle chicken with 1 teaspoon of paprika; brown in kettle until brown on all sides.

3. Add onion and green bell pepper; cook until onions are transparent.

4. Add chicken broth, tomatoes with liquid from can, parsley, Tabasco®, and Worcestershire sauces; bring to a boil.

5. Cover and reduce heat; simmer for 30 minutes.

6. After 30 minutes, add corn and lima beans; cook for an additional 20 minutes.

To serve, divide into 8 equal portions and serve each with equally divided oyster crackers.

*Note: You may also prepare this in a crock pot. Simply place all ingredients into crock pot and cook on medium for six to eight hours.

Nutrition Facts	
Servings Per Meal: 8	
Amount Per Serving	
Calories 340	Calories from Fat 60
Total Fat 7g	
Saturated Fat 1g	
Trans Fat 0g	
Cholesterol 65mg	
Sodium 450mg	
Total Carbohydrate 35g	
Dietary Fiber 5g	
Sugars 6g	
Protein 34g	

Calories Per Gram:
Fat 9 – Carbohydrate 4 – Protein 4

Daily Nutritional Average

Nutrition Facts

Weekly Daily Average

Amount Per Serving

Calories 1200 Calories from Fat 360

Total Fat 40g

Saturated Fat 10.5g

Trans Fat 0g

Cholesterol 215mg

Sodium 1750mg

Total Carbohydrate 120g

Dietary Fiber 19g

Sugars 46g

Protein 89g

Calories Per Gram:
  Fat 9 – Carbohydrate 4 – Protein 4

Week 2 Recipes

Day 8 Autumn Spiced Cottage Cheese and Applesauce
Easy Tuna Casserole
Turkey Marsala Meatballs and Green Bean Stir Fry

Day 9 Creamy Strawberry Banana Yogurt Smoothie
Mexican Chicken Wrap
Pork Tenderloin Diane and Vegetable Medley

Day 10 Pumpkin Pecan Oatmeal and Pears
Skillet Beef and Cheddar Sauté
Poached Salmon with Cucumber Sauce and Parsley Garlic Potatoes

Day 11 Tasty Tomato, Basil, and Cream Cheese Frittata
Shrimp Minted Blueberry Fruit Salad
Tex-Mex Turkey Chili

Day 12 Creamy Peanut Butter Banana Wrap
Mediterranean Greek Salad
Cajun Pork Gumbo Over Couscous

Day 13 Heart Healthy Cheese Filled Honey Crepes
Lemony Chicken Rice
Garlic Shrimp and Pepper Pizza

Day 14 Baked Ham and Eggs Rosemary
Southwestern Chopped Chicken Salad
Sesame Ginger Salmon and Vegetable Bean Antipasto

Week 2 Shopping List

Bread Products

bread crumbs	2 tablespoons
English muffins, whole wheat	3
pita bread, whole wheat	6 small

Canned Beans

black beans, low sodium	1 cup
kidney beans, low sodium	1 cup
navy beans	1 cup

Canned Fruits

applesauce, unsweetened	1/2 cup
mandarin oranges, in juice	3 cups
pears, in juice	2 cups

Canned Seafood & Meat

chicken, in broth	4 5 ounce cans
tuna, in water	10 ounces

Canned Vegetables

pumpkin puree	1/2 cup
tomatoes	16 ounces

Cereals

oats, quick-cooking	1 cup

Dairy Products

Asiago cheese	1/2 ounce
butter	2 tablespoons
butter, unsalted	2 teaspoons
cheddar cheese, sharp, shredded	1 cup
cottage cheese, low-fat	1 cup
cream cheese, light	4 ounces
cream cheese, nonfat	6 ounces
egg whites	2 large
eggs	1 large
feta cheese, reduced fat	7 ounces
margarine, stick	2 tablespoons
milk, 1%	1/2 cup
milk, nonfat	5-1/2 cups
Monterey jack cheese with jalapeno	1/2 cup shredded
mozzarella cheese, part skim	1-1/2 cups shredded
parmesan cheese	1 cup fresh shredded
ricotta cheese, part skim	4 ounces
sour cream, light	1-1/2 cups
yogurt, light vanilla	2 cups

Deli Lunchmeat

ham, lean	4 ounces

Dried Fruit

raisins, golden	2 tablespoons

Fresh Seafood & Fish

salmon	2 pounds
shrimp	2 pounds

Frozen Foods

egg substitute	5 cups
strawberries, unsweetened	3 cups
peas	1-1/2 cups
spinach, chopped	10 ounces

Jams & Jellies

honey	1 tablespoon
natural peanut butter	1 tablespoon

Meat & Poultry

beef, lean ground	1 pound
chicken breasts, boneless/ skinless, pork tenderloin	1 pound 2 pounds
turkey breast, ground	4 pounds

Mexican Food Products

green chilies, canned	1 4 ounce can
tortillas, whole wheat	7 small

Nuts & Seeds

pecans	2 tablespoons
walnuts	2 tablespoons

Oriental Food Products

soy sauce	2 tablespoons

Pasta

couscous, dry	1 cup
elbow macaroni, whole wheat, dry	6 ounces
pasta, whole wheat, dry	8 ounces

Pickles & Olives

black olives, sliced	1/2 cup
Kalamata olives	1/4 cup
pimientos	1/2 cup

Produce

asparagus tips	1 cup
bananas	1 medium
basil leaves, fresh	1 cup
Bibb lettuce	1/2 head
blueberries	1-3/4 cups
broccoli flowerets	1 cup
cantaloupe	1 large
carrots, baby	1 cup
carrots, sliced	1/2 cup
carrots, shredded	2 cups
celery	1 stalk
cherries	6 cups
chives, fresh	1 tablespoon
cilantro, fresh	1 tablespoon
cucumbers	2 medium
garlic	17 cloves
ginger, fresh	3/4 teaspoon
grapes	1 medium bunch
green beans	1 pound
leaf lettuce	2 cups
leeks	1 large
lemon juice	1/2 cup
lemon zest	2 lemons
lime juice	1/4 cup
lime zest	1 large lime
mint leaves, fresh	1/4 cup
mushrooms	1 pound

onions, green	3 bunches
onions, red	1 small
onions, yellow	4 medium
oregano, fresh	1 teaspoon
parsley, fresh	1 bunch
peach	1 large
peppers, green bell	3 medium
peppers, red bell	4 medium
pepper, yellow bell	1 medium
potato	1 medium
potatoes, red	1/2 pound
romaine lettuce	4 leaves
strawberries	1 cup
tomatoes	9 medium
tomatoes, plum	3 medium
summer squash, yellow	1 large
zucchini	1 medium

Salad Dressings

Italian, reduced calorie	1/2 cup

Soups

chicken broth, low sodium	1 cup

Cooking Spirits

Marsala wine	1/2 cup
white wine	3/4 cup

Tomato Sauces

pizza sauce	1/2 cup
tomato paste	2 tablespoons
tomato sauce	8 ounces

Daily Menu

Breakfast

- o Autumn Spiced Cottage Cheese and Applesauce

Mid Morning Snack

- o 125 Calorie Snack

Lunch

- o Easy Tuna Casserole with Mandarin Oranges

Mid Afternoon Snack

- o 100 Calorie Snack

Dinner

- o Turkey Marsala Meatballs and Green Bean Stir Fry

Evening Snack

- o 100 Calorie Snack

Nutrition Facts

Daily Menu

Amount Per Serving

Calories 1200 Calories from Fat 340

Total Fat 38g	
Saturated Fat 8g	
Trans Fat 0g	
Cholesterol 150mg	
Sodium 2375mg	
Total Carbohydrate 132g	
Dietary Fiber 22g	
Sugars 42g	
Protein 83g	

Calories Per Gram:
Fat 9 – Carbohydrate 4 – Protein 4

Breakfast
Autumn Spiced Cottage Cheese and Applesauce

Serves 1

1/2 cup	low-fat cottage cheese
1/4 teaspoon	pumpkin pie spice
1/4 teaspoon	vanilla extract
2 tablespoons	walnuts, chopped
1/2 cup	unsweetened applesauce
1 packet	Splenda®

Directions

1. In a small bowl combine cottage cheese, spice, and vanilla extract; mix well.

2. In another small bowl add applesauce and Splenda®.

3. Mix well into cottage cheese.

4. Garnish cottage cheese with walnuts.

Nutrition Facts
Servings Per Meal: 1

Amount Per Serving

Calories 230　Calories from Fat 100

Total Fat 11g

Saturated Fat 1.5g

Trans Fat 0g

Cholesterol 5mg

Sodium 460mg

Total Carbohydrate 18g

Dietary Fiber 3g

Sugars 13g

Protein 16g

Calories Per Gram:
Fat 9 – Carbohydrate 4 – Protein 4

Lunch
Easy Tuna Casserole
with Mandarin Oranges

Serves 6

6 ounces	whole wheat elbow macaroni, uncooked
2 tablespoons	margarine, divided
8 ounces	mushrooms, sliced
3 tablespoons	all-purpose flour
1 tablespoon	Dijon mustard
1-3/4 cups	nonfat milk
1/4 teaspoon	salt
10 ounces	tuna in water, canned, drained and flaked
2 ounces	pimientos, drained and sliced
1/3 cup	parmesan cheese, grated
1-1/2 cups	frozen peas, defrosted
1 pinch	black pepper, to taste
3 cups	mandarin oranges in juice, drained

Nutrition Facts
Servings Per Meal: 6

Amount Per Serving

Calories 330   Calories from Fat 60

Total Fat 7g

Saturated Fat 2g

Trans Fat 0g

Cholesterol 25mg

Sodium 590mg

Total Carbohydrate 44g

Dietary Fiber 6g

Sugars 14g

Protein 24g

Calories Per Gram:
Fat 9 – Carbohydrate 4 – Protein 4

Directions

1. Preheat oven to 350° F.
2. Prepare pasta according to package directions.
3. While pasta is cooking, melt 1 tablespoon margarine in skillet over medium-high heat.
4. Add mushrooms and sauté 2 to 3 minutes.
5. Drain off any liquid and set mushrooms aside.
6. Place the remaining margarine in the skillet and melt over medium-low heat.
7. With a wire whisk, stir in flour.
8. Gradually add the Dijon mustard, milk and salt, stirring constantly until mixture boils and thickens. Once thickened, stir in mushrooms and remove from heat.
9. When pasta is done, drain well. Return pasta to the pot and add tuna, mushroom mixture, pimentos, cheese, peas, and pepper.
10. Combine all ingredients together and transfer to a 2-quart casserole dish.
11. Bake for 15 minutes or until thoroughly heated.

To serve, divide casserole into 6 equal portions and serve each with 1/2 cup mandarin oranges.

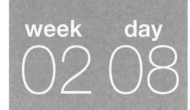

Dinner
Turkey Meatballs Marsala and Green Bean Stir Fry
with Whole Wheat Pasta

Serves 5

Turkey Meatballs Marsala:

2 tablespoons	bread crumbs
2 tablespoons	green onion, chopped
1 teaspoon	dry Marsala wine (for meatballs)
1/4 teaspoon	salt
1/4 teaspoon	black pepper
1 pound	lean ground turkey
1 clove	garlic, minced
2 teaspoons	olive oil
1/2 cup	leek, chopped
1 cup	water
1/2 cup	1% milk
2 tablespoons	golden raisins
1/2 teaspoon	lemon zest
1/4 teaspoon	dried thyme
1/2 cup	dry Marsala wine (for sauce)
1 tablespoon	cornstarch
1/4 teaspoon	salt
1 cup	whole wheat pasta, cooked

Turkey Meatball Marsala Directions

1. Combine first 7 ingredients in a bowl; shape mixture into 25 (1-inch) meatballs.
2. Heat oil in a large nonstick skillet over medium-high heat.
3. Add meatballs; cook 10 minutes or until done.
4. Remove meatballs from pan; set aside.
5. Add leek to pan, and sauté 3 minutes or until tender.
6. Stir in water and next 4 ingredients (water through thyme), and bring to a boil.
7. Combine 1/2 cup Marsala wine, cornstarch, and 1/4 teaspoon salt, stirring with a whisk.
8. Add Marsala mixture to leek mixture; cook over medium heat for 6 minutes or until slightly thick.
9. Return meatballs to pan and cook 3 minutes or until thoroughly heated.

Recipe Continued On Next Page…

Nutrition Facts
Servings Per Meal: 5

Amount Per Serving

Calories 320 Calories from Fat 100

Total Fat 11g
  Saturated Fat 2.5g
  Trans Fat 0g
Cholesterol 75mg
Sodium 530mg
Total Carbohydrate 28g
  Dietary Fiber 4g
  Sugars 8g
Protein 21g

Calories Per Gram:
  Fat 9 – Carbohydrate 4 – Protein 4

Dinner (continued)
Turkey Meatballs Marsala and Green Bean Stir Fry
with Whole Wheat Pasta

Green Bean Stir Fry:

1-1/2 teaspoons	**olive oil**
1 pound	**green beans, cleaned and ends removed**
1 large	**red bell pepper, julienne**
1/2 cup	**yellow summer squash, seeded and sliced**
1 cup	**red onion, sliced thin**
1 clove	**garlic, minced**
1 teaspoon	**salt**
1/2 teaspoon	**red pepper**
1/4 cup	**white wine**
2 tablespoons	**fresh lemon juice**
1 pinch	**salt and pepper**

Green Bean Stir Fry Directions

1. In a large sauté pan over medium high heat add olive oil.

2. Add green beans; sauté for 5 to 7 minutes.

3. Add red pepper, yellow squash, onion, and garlic and sauté over medium heat 4 to 6 minutes.

4. Add white wine to deglaze the pan and reduce wine by half.

5. Add salt, pepper, and lemon juice and toss well.

To serve, divide meatballs and green bean stir fry into 5 equal portions and serve meatballs over pasta.

*Note: You may also prepare this in a crock pot. Simply place all ingredients into crock pot and cook on medium for six to eight hours.

Daily Menu

Breakfast

o Creamy Strawberry Banana Yogurt Smoothie

Mid Morning Snack

o 100 Calorie Snack

Lunch

o Mexican Chicken Wrap

Mid Afternoon Snack

o 100 Calorie Snack

Dinner

o Pork Tenderloin Diane and Vegetable Medley

Evening Snack

o 100 Calorie Snack

Nutrition Facts

Daily Menu

Amount Per Serving

Calories 1200 Calories from Fat 290

Total Fat 32g

 Saturated Fat 9g

 Trans Fat 0g

Cholesterol 190mg

Sodium 2020mg

Total Carbohydrate 140g

 Dietary Fiber 18g

 Sugars 49g

Protein 87g

Calories Per Gram:
 Fat 9 – Carbohydrate 4 – Protein 4

Breakfast
Creamy Strawberry Banana Yogurt Smoothie

Serves 1

1 cup	light vanilla yogurt
1/2 cup	nonfat milk
1/2	medium banana
1 cup	fresh strawberries, sliced

Directions

1. Place all ingredients into blender and blend until smooth.

Nutrition Facts
Servings Per Meal: 1

Amount Per Serving

Calories 270   Calories from Fat 5

Total Fat 1g

Saturated Fat 0g

Trans Fat 0g

Cholesterol 5mg

Sodium 180mg

Total Carbohydrate 53g

Dietary Fiber 5g

Sugars 36g

Protein 13g

Calories Per Gram:
Fat 9 – Carbohydrate 4 – Protein 4

Lunch
Mexican Chicken Wraps

Serves 6

2 medium	tomatoes, chopped
1 4 ounce can	green chilies, diced
1/3 cup	green onions, sliced
1 tablespoon	fresh cilantro, chopped
1 tablespoon	canola oil
1 pound	boneless skinless chicken breast, cut into 1" cubes
2 tablespoons	water
1 ounce	taco seasoning mix*
6 each	whole wheat tortillas
6 tablespoons	light sour cream

Directions

Nutrition Facts
Servings Per Meal: 6
Amount Per Serving
Calories 300   Calories from Fat 70
Total Fat 8g
Saturated Fat 1g
Trans Fat 0g
Cholesterol 50mg
Sodium 590mg
Total Carbohydrate 29g
Dietary Fiber 3g
Sugars 3g
Protein 23g
Calories Per Gram: Fat 9 – Carbohydrate 4 – Protein 4

1. In large bowl, combine tomatoes, chilies, green onions, and cilantro; set aside.

2. In large skillet, heat oil over medium-high heat; add chicken and cook about 2 minutes.

3. Add water and taco seasoning mix; continue to cook until chicken is cooked through.

4. Mix in tomato mixture to skillet of seasoned chicken.

5. Place 1/4 cup filling on each tortilla; roll up.

6. Garnish with 1 tablespoon sour cream.

*Note: Fillings may be prepared the night before, and then wrapped in tortillas the next day.

Dinner
Pork Tenderloin Diane and Vegetable Medley

Serves 4

Pork Tenderloin Diane:

1 pound	lean pork tenderloin, cut into 8 equal pieces*
2 teaspoons	lemon pepper
1 tablespoon	butter
2 tablespoons	fresh lemon juice
1 tablespoon	Worcestershire sauce
1 teaspoon	Dijon mustard
1 tablespoon	chives

Pork Tenderloin Directions

1. Press each tenderloin slice to a 1-in. thickness.

2. Sprinkle surfaces of medallions with lemon pepper.

3. Heat butter in heavy skillet; cook tenderloin medallions 3-4 minutes on each side.

4. Remove medallions to serving platter; keep warm.

5. Add lemon juice, Worcestershire sauce, and mustard to skillet; cook until heated through.

6. Pour sauce over medallions; sprinkle with chives and serve.

*Note: Can also be roasted whole and sliced at meal time.

Recipe Continued On Next Page...

Nutrition Facts	
Servings Per Meal: 4	
Amount Per Serving	
Calories 320 Calories from Fat 130	
Total Fat 14g	
Saturated Fat 6g	
Trans Fat 0g	
Cholesterol 95mg	
Sodium 520mg	
Total Carbohydrate 18g	
Dietary Fiber 4g	
Sugars 5g	
Protein 31g	

Calories Per Gram:
Fat 9 – Carbohydrate 4 – Protein 4

Dinner (continued)
Pork Tenderloin Diane and Vegetable Medley

Vegetable Medley:

1 tablespoon	olive oil
1 cup	baby carrots
1 cup	broccoli florets
1 cup	potatoes, peeled and diced
1 small	red bell pepper, chopped
1 small	yellow bell pepper, chopped
1 cup	yellow squash, sliced
1 cup	zucchini, sliced
1 small	onion, chopped
1 tablespoon	olive oil
1 clove	garlic, minced
2 tablespoons	fresh lemon juice
1/2 cup	parmesan cheese, shredded

Vegetable Medley Directions

1. In a large sauté pan heat oil to medium high heat.

2. Add vegetables and sauté for 7 minutes or until vegetables are soft to the touch.

3. Add lemon juice; sauté one more minute.

4. Top with parmesan cheese.

Breakfast
- o Pumpkin Pecan Oatmeal and Pears

Mid Morning Snack
- o 100 Calorie Snack

Lunch
- o Skillet Beef and Cheddar Sauté

Mid Afternoon Snack
- o 100 Calorie Snack

Dinner
- o Poached Salmon with Cucumber Sauce and Parsley Garlic Potatoes

Evening Snack
- o 75 Calorie Snack

Nutrition Facts
Daily Menu

Amount Per Serving

Calories 1200 Calories from Fat 340

Total Fat 38g	
Saturated Fat 8g	
Trans Fat 0g	
Cholesterol 150mg	
Sodium 2375mg	
Total Carbohydrate 132g	
Dietary Fiber 22g	
Sugars 42g	
Protein 83g	

Calories Per Gram:
Fat 9 – Carbohydrate 4 – Protein 4

Breakfast
Pumpkin Pecan Oatmeal and Pears

Serves 4

1 cup	nonfat milk
1/2 cup	nonfat powdered milk
1/2 teaspoon	pumpkin pie spice
1 cup	quick cooking oats, uncooked
1/2 cup	canned pumpkin puree
2 tablespoons	Splenda®
2 cups	canned pears in juice, diced
8 ounces	light vanilla yogurt
2 tablespoons	pecans, coarsely chopped

Nutrition Facts

Servings Per Meal: *4*

Amount Per Serving

Calories 250   Calories from Fat 40

Total Fat 4.5g

   Saturated Fat 0g

   Trans Fat 0g

Cholesterol 5mg

Sodium 105mg

Total Carbohydrate 43g

   Dietary Fiber 6g

   Sugars 22g

Protein 11g

Calories Per Gram:
Fat 9 – Carbohydrate 4 – Protein 4

Directions

1. In medium saucepan, bring milk, powdered milk, and pie spice to a boil; stir in oats.

2. Return to a boil; reduce heat to medium.

3. Cook 1 minute for quick oats or until most of liquid is absorbed, stirring occasionally.

4. Stir in pumpkin, Splenda®, and pears; cook 1 minute. Let stand until desired consistency.

5. Spoon oatmeal into four cereal bowls.

6. Top with yogurt and pecans.

*Note: No sugar has been added. All sugar is naturally occurring from the fruit and dairy.

Lunch
Skillet Beef and Cheddar Sauté

Serves 6

1 pound	lean ground beef, less than 20% fat
1/2 cup	onion, chopped
1 cup	carrots, shredded
8 ounces	tomato sauce
1/4 cup	pitted ripe olives, halved
4 ounces	whole wheat noodles, uncooked
2 cups	water
1 teaspoon	dried oregano
1/4 teaspoon	black pepper
1/2 cup	sharp cheddar cheese, shredded

Nutrition Facts

Servings Per Meal: 6

Amount Per Serving

Calories 340   Calories from Fat 160

Total Fat 17g

Saturated Fat 7g

Trans Fat 0g

Cholesterol 75mg

Sodium 390mg

Total Carbohydrate 20g

Dietary Fiber 3g

Sugars 3g

Protein 26g

Calories Per Gram:
Fat 9 – Carbohydrate 4 – Protein 4

Directions

1. Cook and stir the meat and onion in a large skillet until the meat is brown.
2. Drain off the excess fat.
3. Stir in the rest of the ingredients.
4. Finish with one of the methods below.

To Cook in a Skillet

1. Heat the mixture to boiling then reduce the heat and simmer, uncovered, stirring occasionally, until the noodles are tender, about 20 minutes.
2. Serve hot.

To Cook in an Oven

1. Preheat oven to 375 F°.
2. Pour the mixture into an ungreased 2-quart casserole.
3. Cover and bake for 30 minutes, stirring occasionally.

Dinner
Poached Salmon with Cucumber Sauce and Parsley Garlic Potatoes
with Asparagus

Serves 4

1 cup	water
1/2 cup	dry white wine
1 small	onion, sliced
2 teaspoons	parsley, chopped
5 each	peppercorns
1/4 teaspoon	salt
1 pound	salmon steaks cut into 4 equal pieces

Salmon Directions

1. In a large sauté pan add the water, wine, onion, parsley, and peppercorns and bring to a light simmer.

2. Once poaching liquid has simmered for 5 minutes add salmon making sure the salmon is covered by the liquid. (If not add more water)

3. Poach for 6-8 minutes depending on thickness of fish.

Cucumber Sauce:

1/2 cup	light sour cream
1/3 cup	cucumber, seeded and finely chopped
1 tablespoon	onion, minced
1/4 teaspoon	salt
1/4 teaspoon	basil, chopped

Recipe continued on next page...

Nutrition Facts

Servings Per Meal: 4

Amount Per Serving

Calories 320   Calories from Fat 150

Total Fat 17g
Saturated Fat 5g
Trans Fat 0g

Cholesterol 80mg

Sodium 540mg

Total Carbohydrate 13g
Dietary Fiber 2g
Sugars 2g

Protein 27g

Calories Per Gram:
Fat 9 – Carbohydrate 4 – Protein 4

Dinner (continued)
Poached Salmon with Cucumber Sauce and Parsley Garlic Potatoes

with Asparagus

Cucumber Sauce Directions

1. Combine sour cream, cucumber, onion, salt, and basil; mix well.

2. Top salmon with cucumber sauce.

Note: Sauce can be made ahead and refrigerated. Yields about 2/3 cup.

Parsley Garlic Potatoes:

1/2 pound	red potatoes, whole, cooked, and drained
2 teaspoons	butter
1 clove	garlic, minced
2 teaspoons	fresh parsley, chopped
1/2 teaspoon	salt
1/4 teaspoon	black pepper
1 cup	asparagus tips, steamed

Parsley Garlic Potatoes Directions

1. In a medium pot bring potatoes to a boil and boil until potatoes are cooked (approx 12 minutes).

2. Drain water from potatoes.

3. Add butter, garlic, parsley, salt and pepper, and mash together with fork until potatoes are just broken apart, yet still in large pieces.

To serve, plate 1 piece of fish with sauce, 2 ounces potatoes, and 1/4 cup asparagus tips.

Breakfast

o Tasty Tomato, Basil, and Cream Cheese Frittata with Grapes

Mid Morning Snack

o 150 Calorie Snack

Lunch

o Shrimp Minted Blueberry Fruit Salad with Whole Wheat English Muffin

Mid Afternoon Snack

o 150 Calorie Snack

Dinner

o Tex-Mex Turkey Chili

Evening Snack

o 100 Calorie Snack

Nutrition Facts
Daily Menu

Amount Per Serving

Calories 1200 Calories from Fat 370

Total Fat 41g

Saturated Fat 10g

Trans Fat 0g

Cholesterol 325mg

Sodium 2215mg

Total Carbohydrate 113g

Dietary Fiber 18g

Sugars 57g

Protein 95g

Calories Per Gram:
Fat 9 – Carbohydrate 4 – Protein 4

Breakfast
Tasty Tomato, Basil, and Cream Cheese Frittata
with Grapes

Serves 6

3 cups	egg substitute
1/4 teaspoon	dried sage
1/4 teaspoon	dried oregano
1/4 teaspoon	dried thyme
1 teaspoon	butter
3 medium	plum tomatoes, sliced
1 cup	fresh basil leaves, finely chopped
6 ounces	fat-free cream cheese, cubed
3 cups	grapes

Nutrition Facts	
Servings Per Meal: 6	
Amount Per Serving	
Calories 210	Calories from Fat 50
Total Fat 5g	
Saturated Fat 1.5g	
Trans Fat 0g	
Cholesterol 5mg	
Sodium 390mg	
Total Carbohydrate 22g	
Dietary Fiber 2g	
Sugars 17g	
Protein 20g	
Calories Per Gram: Fat 9 – Carbohydrate 4 – Protein 4	

Directions

1. Whisk together egg substitute, salt, pepper, sage, oregano, and thyme.

2. In large skillet, melt butter over medium heat; add tomatoes and sauté one minute.

3. Lower heat and add basil, sautéing until limp, 1-2 minutes.

4. Pour egg mixture over all and top with cream cheese cubes.

5. Cover and cook over low heat approximately 20 minutes or until set on top; or cook until bottom is partially set and finish cooking top under broiler.

To serve, divide frittata into 6 equal portions and serve each with 1/2 cup grapes.

Lunch
Shrimp Minted Blueberry Fruit Salad
with Whole Wheat English Muffin

Serves 6

1-3/4 cups	fresh blueberries
1 large	peach, peeled, pitted, and sliced
2 cups	cantaloupe, diced
1/2 head	Bibb lettuce, torn into bite size pieces
1 pound	shrimp, cooked and peeled

Creamy Mint Dressing:

1/4 cup	fresh mint leaves, chopped
3 tablespoons	canola oil
1/4 cup	lime juice
2 tablespoons	Splenda®
1/2 teaspoon	lime zest

3	whole wheat English muffins, cut in half

Directions

1.   Place all ingredients into a large mixing bowl and toss until mixed well.

To serve, divide shrimp salad into 6 equal portions and serve each with 1/2 whole wheat English muffin.

*Note: No sugar has been added. All sugar is naturally occurring from the fruit and dairy.

Dinner
Tex-Mex Turkey Chili

Serves 8

2 pounds	lean ground turkey
1 tablespoon	olive oil
16 ounces	canned tomatoes, chopped
2 cups	onion, chopped
3 cloves	garlic, chopped
3/4 teaspoon	salt
1 tablespoon	chili powder
1 teaspoon	ground cumin
1/2 teaspoon	dried oregano
1/2 teaspoon	black pepper
1 each	bay leaf
1 cup	canned reduced sodium kidney beans
8 tablespoons	light sour cream
8 tablespoons	sharp cheddar cheese, shredded

Nutrition Facts
Servings Per Meal: 8

Amount Per Serving

Calories 300   Calories from Fat 140

Total Fat 15g

Saturated Fat 5g

Trans Fat 0g

Cholesterol 100mg

Sodium 510mg

Total Carbohydrate 14g

Dietary Fiber 3g

Sugars 4g

Protein 25g

Calories Per Gram:
Fat 9 – Carbohydrate 4 – Protein 4

Directions

1. In a large sauté pan, brown turkey in oil, stirring frequently.

2. Add undrained tomatoes, onions, garlic, salt, and remaining seasonings.

3. Cover and simmer for 45 minutes.

4. Stir in kidney beans.

5. Cook for an additional 30 minutes; remove bay leaf.

To serve, divide into 8 equal portions and garnish each with 1 tablespoon cheese and 1 tablespoon light sour cream.

Breakfast

- o Creamy Peanut Butter Banana Wrap with Cottage Cheese

Mid Morning Snack

- o 125 Calorie Snack

Lunch

- o Mediterranean Greek Salad

Mid Afternoon Snack

- o 125 Calorie Snack

Dinner

- o Cajun Pork Gumbo Over Couscous

Evening Snack

- o 50 Calorie Snack

Nutrition Facts
Daily Menu

Amount Per Serving

Calories 1200 Calories from Fat 390

Total Fat 43g

Saturated Fat 9g

Trans Fat 0g

Cholesterol 160mg

Sodium 2130mg

Total Carbohydrate 110g

Dietary Fiber 16g

Sugars 40g

Protein 94g

Calories Per Gram:
Fat 9 – Carbohydrate 4 – Protein 4

Breakfast
Creamy Peanut Butter Banana Wrap
with Cottage Cheese

Serves 1

1 small	**whole wheat tortilla**
1 tablespoon	**natural peanut butter**
1/2	**banana, cut lengthwise**
1/2 cup	**1% cottage cheese**

Directions

1. Spread peanut butter over top of tortilla, add banana, and roll up.

2. Serve cottage cheese on the side.

Nutrition Facts

Servings Per Meal: 1

Amount Per Serving

Calories 300   Calories from Fat 100

Total Fat 11g

   Saturated Fat 2g

   Trans Fat 0g

Cholesterol 5mg

Sodium 600mg

Total Carbohydrate 31g

   Dietary Fiber 4g

   Sugars 12g

Protein 20g

Calories Per Gram:
  Fat 9 – Carbohydrate 4 – Protein 4

Lunch
Mediterranean Greek Salad

Serves 4

3/4 pound	99% fat-free ground turkey
2 cloves	garlic, minced
1 teaspoon	dried oregano
1/4 teaspoon	cumin

Directions

1. Heat medium non stick pan; add turkey, garlic, dried oregano, and cumin; sauté until turkey is cooked to 165° F (10 to 15 minutes).

Dressing:

3 tablespoons	olive oil
2 tablespoons	fresh lemon juice
1 tablespoon	red wine vinegar
1 teaspoon	garlic, minced
1 teaspoon	fresh oregano, chopped

Ingredients:

1/4 cup	Kalamata olives
1 large	cucumber, peeled and chopped
1 tablespoon	fresh parsley, chopped
6 large	green onions, sliced
1 dash	black pepper, to taste
4 leaves	romaine lettuce
3 ounces	reduced fat feta cheese
2 medium	tomatoes, cut into wedges

Dressing Directions

1. Whisk together olive oil, lemon juice, vinegar, garlic, and oregano.
2. Combine the olives, cucumbers, chopped parsley and green onions in a bowl; add dressing.
3. Toss to mix; season to taste with pepper.
4. Line plates or a platter with the romaine lettuce leaves.
5. Add the olive-cucumber mixture and sprinkle the feta cheese.
6. Garnish as desired with cooked seasoned turkey and tomato wedges.

Nutrition Facts	
Servings Per Meal: 4	
Amount Per Serving	
Calories 290	Calories from Fat 150
Total Fat 17g	
Saturated Fat 3.5g	
Trans Fat 0g	
Cholesterol 40mg	
Sodium 490mg	
Total Carbohydrate 10g	
Dietary Fiber 2g	
Sugars 4g	
Protein 27g	

Calories Per Gram:
Fat 9 – Carbohydrate 4 – Protein 4

Dinner
Cajun Pork Gumbo Over Couscous

Serves 4

1 pound	lean pork tenderloin
2/3 cup	low sodium chicken broth
2 tablespoons	tomato paste
1 tablespoon	cornstarch
1 teaspoon	dried thyme, crushed
1/4 teaspoon	ground red pepper
1/4 teaspoon	black pepper
1/4 teaspoon	salt
1 tablespoon	canola oil
3/4 cup	celery, sliced
1/2 cup	onion, chopped
3 cloves	garlic, minced
1 medium	green bell pepper, seeded and chopped
3 medium	tomatoes, seeded and chopped
2 cups	couscous, cooked

Nutrition Facts
Servings Per Meal: 4

Amount Per Serving

Calories 320   Calories from Fat 70

Total Fat 8g

   Saturated Fat 1.5g

   Trans Fat 0g

Cholesterol 75mg

Sodium 310mg

Total Carbohydrate 32g

   Dietary Fiber 4g

   Sugars 6g

Protein 30g

Calories Per Gram:
Fat 9 – Carbohydrate 4 – Protein 4

Directions

1. Partially freeze pork tenderloin (this makes it easier to slice).
2. Thinly slice pork into bite-sized strips; set aside.
3. Combine broth, tomato paste, cornstarch, thyme, red pepper, black pepper, and salt; set aside.
4. Preheat a large sauté pan.
5. Add oil, swirling to coat pan.
6. Add pork strips; quickly stir to spread evenly.
7. Sauté for 4-5 minutes; remove meat from pan.
8. Add celery, onion, and garlic to pan.
9. Sauté for 3-4 minutes or until tender.
10. Stir in green pepper, chopped tomato, and broth mixture.
11. Cover and simmer over medium heat for 5 minutes. Gumbo will be slightly thickened and bubbly. Stir in pork.
12. Serve over couscous.

Daily Menu

Breakfast

o Heart Healthy Cheese Filled Honey Crepes with Strawberries

Mid Morning Snack

o 100 Calorie Snack

Lunch

o Lemony Chicken Rice

Mid Afternoon Snack

o 100 Calorie Snack

Dinner

o Garlic Shrimp and Pepper Pizza

Evening Snack

o 100 Calorie Snack

Nutrition Facts
Daily Menu
Amount Per Serving
Calories 1200 Calories from Fat 325
Total Fat 36g
Saturated Fat 13g
Trans Fat 0g
Cholesterol 295mg
Sodium 1760mg
Total Carbohydrate 126g
Dietary Fiber 17g
Sugars 35g
Protein 92g

Calories Per Gram:
Fat 9 – Carbohydrate 4 – Protein 4

Breakfast
Heart Healthy Cheese Filled Honey Crepes
with Strawberries

Serves 6

2 cups	nonfat milk
1 cup	all-purpose flour
2 large	egg whites
1 large	egg
1 tablespoon	honey
1 tablespoon	canola oil
1/8 teaspoon	salt

Crepe Directions

1. Combine all ingredients in a blender; blend until smooth.
2. Rub an 8-inch nonstick skillet with an oiled paper towel, or spray lightly with nonstick cooking spray; heat over medium-high heat.
3. Spoon 4 tablespoons crepe batter into skillet, tilting and rotating skillet to cover evenly with batter.
4. Cook until edges begin to brown.
5. Turn crepe over and cook until lightly browned.
6. Remove crepe to plate to cool.
7. Repeat process with remaining batter.

Crepe Cheese Filling:

4 ounces	part skim ricotta cheese
4 ounces	light cream cheese, softened
1/2 teaspoon	vanilla extract
1/2 teaspoon	cinnamon
3 tablespoons	Splenda®
3 cups	strawberries, unsweetened, thawed

Cheese Filling Directions

1. Place all ingredients into a large mixing bowl, and mix for 2 minutes or until mixture is smooth.
2. Divide cheese mixture evenly over crepes and roll-up.

Serve 1 crepe per person and top with 1/2 cup thawed strawberries per person.

Nutrition Facts

Servings Per Meal: 6

Amount Per Serving

Calories 250   Calories from Fat 70

Total Fat 8g

Saturated Fat 3.5g

Trans Fat 0g

Cholesterol 50mg

Sodium 190mg

Total Carbohydrate 35g

Dietary Fiber 3g

Sugars 13g

Protein 12g

Calories Per Gram:
Fat 9 – Carbohydrate 4 – Protein 4

Lunch
Lemony Chicken Rice

Serves 6

2 tablespoons	olive oil
1-1/2 pounds	boneless skinless chicken breast
1 clove	garlic, minced
1 cup	brown rice, uncooked
3 cups	low sodium chicken broth
1-1/2 cups	frozen green peas
1/4 cup	pimentos
3 tablespoons	lemon juice

Directions

1. Place olive oil into a medium pot and bring to a medium heat.

2. When oil is heated add chicken and garlic; sauté for 2 minutes.

3. Add brown rice and sauté for an additional 1 minute.

4. Add chicken broth, peas, and pimentos; bring to a simmer.

5. Place lid on pot and simmer for 25 minutes or until rice is tender.

6. Add lemon juice.

Nutrition Facts
Servings Per Meal: 6

Amount Per Serving

Calories 330   Calories from Fat 70

Total Fat 8g

   Saturated Fat 1.5g

   Trans Fat 0g

Cholesterol 65mg

Sodium 240mg

Total Carbohydrate 32g

   Dietary Fiber 3g

   Sugars 3g

Protein 33g

Calories Per Gram:
Fat 9 – Carbohydrate 4 – Protein 4

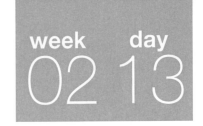
Dinner
Garlic Shrimp and Pepper Pizza

Serves 6

1 pound	medium shrimp, uncooked, peeled, and deveined
1 teaspoon	olive oil
2 cloves	garlic, minced
1/4 cup	red bell pepper, cut into thin strips
1/4 cup	yellow bell pepper, cut into thin strips
1/4 cup	green bell pepper, cut into thin strips
6 small	whole wheat pita bread
1/2 cup	pizza sauce
1-1/2 cups	part skim milk mozzarella cheese, shredded
1/2 ounce	Asiago cheese, shredded

Directions

1. Preheat oven to 450° F.

2. Stir-fry shrimp in oil with garlic in a large skillet over medium-high heat 2 minutes.

3. Add pepper strips; continue to stir-fry 1 to 2 minutes or until shrimp are cooked through; remove from heat.

4. Place pita bread on baking sheet.

5. Spread pizza sauce evenly over pita; add shrimp and peppers.

6. Top with mozzarella and Asiago cheeses.

7. Bake 12 to 14 minutes or until cheese is melted and crust is golden brown.

8. Cut each into 6 wedges.

Nutrition Facts

Servings Per Meal: 6

Amount Per Serving

Calories 300   Calories from Fat 100

Total Fat 11g

Saturated Fat 6g

Trans Fat 0g

Cholesterol 140mg

Sodium 600mg

Total Carbohydrate 20g

Dietary Fiber 4g

Sugars 1g

Protein 27g

Calories Per Gram:
Fat 9 – Carbohydrate 4 – Protein 4

Daily Menu

Breakfast
o Baked Ham and Eggs Rosemary with Cherries

Mid Morning Snack
o 125 Calorie Snack

Lunch
o Southwestern Chopped Chicken Salad

Mid Afternoon Snack
o 125 Calorie Snack

Dinner
o Sesame Ginger Salmon and Vegetable Bean Antipasto

Evening Snack
o 100 Calorie Snack

Nutrition Facts
Daily Menu

Amount Per Serving

Calories 1200 Calories from Fat 400

Total Fat 44g

Saturated Fat 11g

Trans Fat 0g

Cholesterol 175mg

Sodium 2400mg

Total Carbohydrate 109g

Dietary Fiber 23g

Sugars 53g

Protein 91g

Calories Per Gram:
Fat 9 – Carbohydrate 4 – Protein 4

Breakfast
Baked Ham and Eggs Rosemary
with Cherries

Serves 6

1/2 cup	lean ham, cubed
1 10 ounce	package frozen chopped spinach, thawed, and drained well
2 teaspoons	unsalted butter, melted
1-1/2 cups	egg substitute
4 ounces	reduced fat feta cheese
1 teaspoon	crushed rosemary
1 dash	black pepper, to taste
6 cups	cherries

Directions

1. Preheat oven to 350° F.

2. Spray 8 x 8 inch baking dish with nonstick cooking spray.

3. Add ham and top with spinach.

4. Melt butter and brush over spinach.

5. Pour egg substitute over spinach and ham.

6. Sprinkle feta cheese evenly over egg substitute; sprinkle with rosemary and pepper.

7. Bake 20 minutes or until set.

To serve, divide into 6 equal portions and serve with 1 cup cherries.

Nutrition Facts
Servings Per Meal: 6

Amount Per Serving

Calories 220   Calories from Fat 70

Total Fat 8g

Saturated Fat 3g

Trans Fat 0g

Cholesterol 15mg

Sodium 520mg

Total Carbohydrate 26g

Dietary Fiber 4g

Sugars 17g

Protein 17g

Calories Per Gram:
Fat 9 – Carbohydrate 4 – Protein 4

Lunch
Southwestern Chopped Chicken Salad

Serves 6

2 cups	chicken, canned, drained
2 cups	leaf lettuce, chopped
8 ounces	fresh mushrooms, sliced
2 medium	tomatoes, chopped
1 cup	carrot, shredded
1 cup	canned low sodium black beans
1 medium	cucumber, peeled and chopped
1/2 cup	jalapeno cheese, shredded
1/4 cup	pitted black olives, sliced
1/2 cup	low calorie Italian salad dressing
1/2 teaspoon	chili powder

Directions

1. Combine all ingredients in a medium bowl.

2. Divide into 6 equal servings.

Nutrition Facts
Servings Per Meal: 6

Amount Per Serving

Calories 260   Calories from Fat 120

Total Fat 13g

Saturated Fat 4g

Trans Fat 0g

Cholesterol 40mg

Sodium 580mg

Total Carbohydrate 14g

Dietary Fiber 4g

Sugars 4g

Protein 23g

Calories Per Gram:
Fat 9 – Carbohydrate 4 – Protein 4

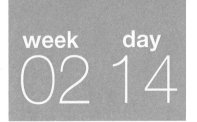

Dinner
Sesame Ginger Salmon
and Vegetable Bean Antipasto

Serves 4

1 pound	salmon, cut into 4 equal pieces
1 tablespoon	sesame oil
2 tablespoons	soy sauce
2 tablespoons	balsamic vinegar
2 tablespoons	green onions, chopped
2 tablespoons	brown sugar
1 clove	garlic, minced
3/4 teaspoon	ginger, grated
1/2 teaspoon	red pepper flakes

Sesame Ginger Salmon Directions

1. Place salmon steaks in glass dish.

2. Whisk together remaining ingredients; pour over salmon.

3. Cover with plastic wrap and marinate in refrigerator 4 hours.

4. Remove salmon from marinade and place on well-oiled grill 5 inches from coals.

5. Grill for 10 minutes per inch of thickness or until fish flakes when tested with a fork. Turn halfway through cooking.

Recipe Continued on Next Page...

Nutrition Facts

Servings Per Meal: 4

Amount Per Serving

Calories 320   Calories from Fat 120

Total Fat 14g

Saturated Fat 2g

Trans Fat 0g

Cholesterol 75mg

Sodium 380mg

Total Carbohydrate 21g

Dietary Fiber 6g

Sugars 8g

Protein 28g

Calories Per Gram:
Fat 9 – Carbohydrate 4 – Protein 4

Dinner (continued)
Sesame Ginger Salmon
with *Vegetable Bean Antipasto*

Vegetable Bean Antipasto:

2 teaspoons	canola oil
1/2 medium	onion, diced
1 medium	red bell pepper, seeded and diced
1 medium	green bell pepper, seeded and diced
1/2 cup	carrots, diced
1/2 cup	green beans, chopped
1-1/2 teaspoons	garlic, minced
2/3 cup	water
1 tablespoon	cider vinegar
1/4 cup	tomato paste
2/3 cup	navy beans, canned, drained
2 tablespoons	parsley, finely chopped

Vegetable Bean Antipasto Directions

1. In a large saucepan, heat the oil over medium heat.

2. Sauté the onion, peppers, carrots, and green beans, stirring occasionally until tender (about 10 minutes).

3. Add the garlic; cook another minute.

4. Add the water, vinegar, tomato paste; simmer covered for 15 minutes.

5. Stir in the beans and salt; garnish with parsley.

Daily Nutritional Average

Nutrition Facts
Weekly Daily Average

Amount Per Serving

Calories 1200 Calories from Fat 315

Total Fat 35g

    Saturated Fat 6.5g

    Trans Fat 0g

Cholesterol 200mg

Sodium 1930mg

Total Carbohydrate 134g

    Dietary Fiber 21g

    Sugars 46g

Protein 87g

Calories Per Gram:
   Fat 9 – Carbohydrate 4 – Protein 4

Week 3 Recipes

Day 15   Sunshine Breakfast Stir Fry
Black Bean Wrap
One Pot Beef Stew

Day 16   Cheddar, Bacon, and Potato Breakfast Bake
Cool Salmon Ranch Salad
Balsamic Glazed Pork Tenderloin and Red Pepper Grits

Day 17   Cinnamon Cottage Cheese and Banana
Chicken Dijon Green Bean and Potato Salad
Easy Scallop Bake

Day 18   Vanilla Whole Grain Pancakes
Quickie Albacore Tuna Salad
Hearty Turkey Lasagna Rolls

Day 19   Ricotta Raspberry Vanilla Whip
Asian Shrimp Pasta Salad
Turkey Apple Rice Stir Fry

Day 20   Banana Bran Muffins
Caribbean Chicken Salad
Beef Ratatouille

Day 21   Cheesy Spinach Cilantro Omelet
Savory Seafood Soup
Roasted Root Vegetables and Pork

Day 22   Pear Spiced Oatmeal Bread Pudding*
White Bean and Chicken Chili
Angel Hair with Sesame Shrimp Sauce

*Extra day in week 3 to accommodate 30 full days of recipes.

Week 3 Shopping List

Baking Products
Splenda®   3 cups

Bread Products
bread, whole wheat   10 slices

Canned Beans
black beans, low sodium   1/2 cup
white beans   2 cups

Canned Fruits
applesauce, unsweetened   1 cup
pears, in juice   2 cups
pineapple, crushed, juice pack   8 ounces

Canned Seafood & Meat
chicken, in broth   6 5 ounce cans
salmon, low sodium   8 ounces
tuna, in water   12 ounces

Canned Vegetables
green beans   1-1/2 cups
potatoes   1 cup
red pepper, roasted   7 ounces
tomatoes   4 14 ounce cans
tomatoes, low sodium   28 ounces
tomatoes, pureed   16 ounces

Cereals
Grape Nut Flakes   6 cups
grits, quick-cooking dry   3/4 cup
oats, quick-cooking   3/4 cup
Shredded Wheat   1 cup
wheat germ   1/2 cup

Condiments
chili sauce   1 teaspoon
chutney   2 tablespoons

Cooking Oils
sesame oil   2 tablespoons

Deli Lunchmeat
Canadian bacon   4 ounces

Dairy Products
butter   3 tablespoons
buttermilk, low-fat   1 quart
cheddar cheese, sharp   1/2 cup shredded
cottage cheese, low-fat   1 cup
cream cheese, light   2 ounces
egg whites   6 large
eggs   6 large
margarine, light tub   1/4 cup
milk, nonfat   5 cups
Monterey jack cheese   1/4 cup shredded
mozzarella cheese, part skim   1/2 cup shredded
ricotta cheese, part skim   3/4 cup
sour cream, light   1 tablespoon
yogurt, nonfat plain   1/2 cup

Dried Beans & Rice
brown rice, dry   2 cups

Dried Fruit
raisins   2 tablespoons

Flours
whole wheat flour   5 cups
whole wheat pastry flour   1-3/4 cups

Fresh Seafood & Fish
scallops   1-1/2 pounds
shrimp   3 pounds

Frozen Foods
egg substitute   3-1/2 cups
corn, baby   1/2 cup
green beans   1 cup
peas   1-1/2 cups
spinach, chopped   3/4 cup

Jams & Jellies
honey   2 tablespoons
natural peanut butter   1 cup
pancake syrup, sugar free   1 cup

Meat & Poultry

beef tenderloin	3/4 pound
beef, lean	1-1/2 pounds
chicken breasts, boneless skinless	3/4 pound
pork tenderloin	2 pounds
turkey breast cutlets	1-1/2 pounds
turkey breast, ground	1 pound

Mexican Food Products

tortillas, whole wheat	1 small

Nuts & Seeds

almonds	2/3 cup
sesame seeds	1 teaspoon
sesame seeds, toasted	2 tablespoons
walnuts	1/4 cup

Oriental Food Products

Japanese soba noodles	1/2 cup
soy sauce, low sodium	1/3 cup
teriyaki sauce	2 teaspoons

Pasta

pasta, whole wheat, angel hair, dry	8 ounces
pasta, whole wheat, lasagna, dry	12 ounces
pasta, whole wheat, shell, dry	1/2 cup

Pickles & Olives

pimientos	2 tablespoons

Produce

apples	3 medium
asparagus tips	1 pound
bananas	7 medium
bean sprouts, fresh	1/2 cup
carrots	1-1/2 pounds
celery	1 stalk
cherries	1 cup
cilantro, fresh	5 tablespoons
cucumber	1 medium
dill, fresh	1 tablespoon
eggplant	1 small
garlic	26 cloves
ginger, fresh	1 tablespoon
grapes	1/2 cup
jalapeno chili peppers	2
lemon juice	1/3 cup
lime juice	3 tablespoons
mixed salad greens	2 cups
mushrooms	12 ounces
onions, green	2 bunches
onions, red	1 medium
onions, yellow	4 medium
onions, yellow	5 large
parsley, fresh	1 bunch
peppers, green bell	4 medium
peppers, red bell	5 medium
pepper, yellow bell	1 small
plums	8 large
potatoes	1-1/4 pounds
raspberries	1 cup
romaine lettuce	1 head
snow peas	1/2 cup
spinach leaves, fresh	2 cups
thyme, fresh	1/4 teaspoon
tomatoes	6 large
zucchini	1 medium

Salad Dressings

ranch salad dressing, reduced fat	4 tablespoons

Snack Foods

graham crackers	4 squares
oyster crackers	1-1/2 cups
whole wheat crackers	16

Soups

chicken broth, low sodium	8 cups

Spirits for Cooking

red wine	3/4 cup
white wine	1/2 cup

Tomato Sauces

tomato paste	6 ounces
tomato paste, low sodium	8 ounces
tomato puree	16 ounces
tomato puree, unsalted	16 ounces

Breakfast
- o Sunshine Breakfast Stir Fry

Mid Morning Snack
- o 125 Calorie Snack

Lunch
- o Black Bean Wrap with Cherries

Mid Afternoon Snack
- o 100 Calorie Snack

Dinner
- o One Pot Beef Stew

Evening Snack
- o 100 Calorie Snack

Nutrition Facts	
Daily Menu	
Amount Per Serving	
Calories 1200	Calories from Fat 280
Total Fat 31g	
Saturated Fat 7g	
Trans Fat 0g	
Cholesterol 144mg	
Sodium 2135mg	
Total Carbohydrate 147g	
Dietary Fiber 26g	
Sugars 57g	
Protein 84g	

Calories Per Gram:
Fat 9 – Carbohydrate 4 – Protein 4

Breakfast
Sunshine Breakfast Stir Fry

Serves 2

1 teaspoon	canola oil
3 large	egg whites
1/2 cup	canned chicken, drained
2 teaspoons	fresh ginger, slivered
1	green onion, thinly sliced
1/2 cup	snow peas
1/2 cup	baby corn
1/2 cup	soba noodles, cooked
1 medium	tomato, sliced
1 tablespoon	low sodium soy sauce
1 tablespoon	cilantro, minced

Nutrition Facts

Nutrition Facts

Servings Per Meal: 2

Amount Per Serving

Calories 270   Calories from Fat 90

Total Fat 10g

   Saturated Fat 2g

   Trans Fat 0g

Cholesterol 25mg

Sodium 480mg

Total Carbohydrate 23g

   Dietary Fiber 3g

   Sugars 5g

Protein 23g

Calories Per Gram:
Fat 9 – Carbohydrate 4 – Protein 4

Directions

1. Add 1 teaspoon oil to sauté pan over medium heat.

2. Add egg whites, cooking lightly into an omelet; remove from heat and slice into strips.

3. Add chicken, ginger, green onions, baby corn, and snow peas.

4. Cook over medium heat until ginger is fragrant and snow peas turn bright green, about 1 minute. Add noodles; sauté, stirring constantly until warm.

5. Add egg strips, tomatoes and soy sauce; stir over heat until hot.

6. Before serving, sprinkle each serving with chopped cilantro.

Lunch
Black Bean Wrap
with Cherries

Serves 1

1/2 cup	**canned low sodium black beans, drained**
1 tablespoon	**light sour cream**
2 tablespoons	**salsa**
1 small	**whole wheat tortilla**
1 cup	**cherries**

Directions

1. In a small bowl mix black beans, light sour cream, and salsa.

2. Cover with plastic wrap and microwave for 2 minutes or until mixture is heated.

3. Spread mixture on tortilla and fold in half.

Serve with 1 cup cherries on the side.

Nutrition Facts
Servings Per Meal: 1

Amount Per Serving

Calories 330   Calories from Fat 40

Total Fat 4.5g

  Saturated Fat 1g

  Trans Fat 0g

Cholesterol 5mg

Sodium 560mg

Total Carbohydrate 65g

  Dietary Fiber 11g

  Sugars 23g

Protein 12g

Calories Per Gram:
Fat 9 – Carbohydrate 4 – Protein 4

Dinner
One Pot Beef Stew

Serves 6

1-1/2 pounds	lean beef, cut into cubes
3 cups	onion, chopped
2 cups	carrots, peeled and sliced
1 cup	red bell pepper, cut into 1/2 inch strips
8 ounces	fresh mushrooms, cleaned
2 medium	tomatoes, chopped
1/2 cup	red wine
1 each	bay leaf
1/4 cup	fresh parsley, chopped
1/4 teaspoon	hot red pepper flakes
1/2 teaspoon	salt
1/4 teaspoon	black pepper
1/2 cup	frozen peas, thawed

Nutrition Facts

Servings Per Meal: 6

Amount Per Serving

Calories 260   Calories from Fat 70

Total Fat 8g

  Saturated Fat 2.5g

  Trans Fat 0g

Cholesterol 65mg

Sodium 300mg

Total Carbohydrate 18g

  Dietary Fiber 4g

  Sugars 9g

Protein 27g

Calories Per Gram:
Fat 9 – Carbohydrate 4 – Protein 4

Directions

1. In a large heavy pot, combine beef, onion, carrots, red pepper, mushrooms, tomatoes, wine, bay leaf, parsley, and red pepper flakes.

2. Cover and simmer over low heat for 1-1/2 hours, stirring occasionally.

3. Stir in salt and black pepper.

4. Cover and cook 10 minutes, stirring occasionally.

5. Add peas and stir to mix.

Note: For crock pot cooking, place all ingredients into slow cooker and let cook for 6 to 8 hours on medium.

Breakfast

o Cheddar, Bacon, and Potato Breakfast Bake

Mid Morning Snack

o 100 Calorie Snack

Lunch

o Cool Salmon Ranch Salad

Mid Afternoon Snack

o 100 Calorie Snack

Dinner

o Balsamic Glazed Pork Tenderloin and Red Pepper Grits

Evening Snack

o 100 Calorie Snack

Nutrition Facts		
Daily Menu		
Amount Per Serving		
Calories 1200 Calories from Fat 360		
Total Fat 40g		
Saturated Fat 14g		
Trans Fat 0g		
Cholesterol 230mg		
Sodium 1970mg		
Total Carbohydrate 113g		
Dietary Fiber 14g		
Sugars 46g		
Protein 95g		

Calories Per Gram:
Fat 9 – Carbohydrate 4 – Protein 4

Breakfast
Cheddar, Bacon, and Potato Breakfast Bake

Serves 4

4 ounces	Canadian bacon, diced
1/2 small	green bell pepper, diced
1/2 small	red bell pepper, diced
1 small	onion, chopped
1 cup	egg substitute
1/2 pound	russet potatoes, peeled and grated
1/2 cup	sharp cheddar cheese, shredded
1/2 teaspoon	black pepper
1 pinch	salt, to taste

Directions

1. Preheat oven to 350° F.

2. Spray a large quiche dish or 4 individual ramekins with nonstick cooking spray.

3. Sauté Canadian bacon, peppers and onion until soft; drain on paper towels.

4. Whisk egg substitute with potatoes, cheese, salt, and pepper.

5. Mix in Canadian bacon and vegetable mixture.

6. Pour into prepared pan spreading mixture evenly.

7. Bake for 45 minutes, until center is set or knife inserted in center comes out clean.

Nutrition Facts
Servings Per Meal: 4

Amount Per Serving

Calories 220   Calories from Fat 70

Total Fat 8g

Saturated Fat 2g

Trans Fat 0g

Cholesterol 15mg

Sodium 660mg

Total Carbohydrate 26g

Dietary Fiber 3g

Sugars 11g

Protein 13g

Calories Per Gram:
Fat 9 – Carbohydrate 4 – Protein 4

Lunch
Cool Salmon Ranch Salad

Serves 2

1 cup	romaine lettuce, chopped
1/2 cup	onion, chopped
1/2 cup	tomato, chopped
1/2 cup	cucumber, peeled and chopped
1/2 cup	red bell pepper, chopped
1 cup	tart apple, peeled and chopped
1 teaspoon	fresh cilantro, chopped
8 ounces	low sodium canned salmon, drained
4 tablespoons	ranch salad dressing, low-fat
1 pinch	salt and pepper, to taste

Directions

1. Mix chopped vegetables and apple together in mixing bowl.

2. Combine remaining ingredients.

3. Pour over vegetables and apple.

4. Toss and serve.

Nutrition Facts
Servings Per Meal: 2

Amount Per Serving

Calories 290   Calories from Fat 100

Total Fat 12g

Saturated Fat 2g

Trans Fat 0g

Cholesterol 65mg

Sodium 320mg

Total Carbohydrate 23g

Dietary Fiber 4g

Sugars 13g

Protein 25g

Calories Per Gram:
Fat 9 – Carbohydrate 4 – Protein 4

Dinner

Balsamic Glazed Pork Tenderloin and Red Pepper Grits

Serves 4

3 cups	low sodium chicken broth
3/4 cup	quick cooking grits, uncooked
2 tablespoons	butter
1 clove	garlic, minced
7 ounces	roasted red peppers, drained and diced
1 coat	cooking spray
1 pound	lean pork tenderloin, cut into 4 equal portions
1/8 teaspoon	black pepper
1/4 cup	balsamic vinegar
2 tablespoons	honey

Nutrition Facts

Servings Per Meal: *4*

Amount Per Serving

Calories 380   Calories from Fat 100

Total Fat 11g

Saturated Fat 5g

Trans Fat 0g

Cholesterol 90mg

Sodium 290mg

Total Carbohydrate 39g

Dietary Fiber 1g

Sugars 13g

Protein 31g

Calories Per Gram:
Fat 9 – Carbohydrate 4 – Protein 4

Directions

1. Bring broth to a boil.
2. Add grits, butter, and garlic, stirring with a whisk.
3. Reduce heat and simmer, uncovered, for 5 minutes.
4. Remove from heat; stir in red pepper. Cover and set aside.
5. While grits sit, heat a large nonstick skillet coated with cooking spray over medium-high heat.
6. Sprinkle pork with black pepper.
7. Add pork to pan; cook 4 minutes on each side or until done.
8. Remove from pan.
9. Stir in vinegar and honey, scraping pan to loosen browned bits.
10. Bring to a boil; cook 1 minute or until thick, stirring constantly with a whisk.
11. Return pork to pan; turn to coat.

To serve, divide grits into 4 equal portions and place on a plate. Add 1 piece of pork and evenly divide sauce over grits.

Daily Menu

Breakfast

o Cinnamon Cottage Cheese and Banana with Shredded Wheat

Mid Morning Snack

o 125 Calorie Snack

Lunch

o Chicken Dijon Green Bean and Potato Salad

Mid Afternoon Snack

o 100 Calorie Snack

Dinner

o Easy Scallop Bake

Evening Snack

o 100 Calorie Snack

Nutrition Facts	
Daily Menu	
Amount Per Serving	
Calories 1200	Calories from Fat 270
Total Fat 30g	
Saturated Fat 7g	
Trans Fat 0g	
Cholesterol 125mg	
Sodium 2085mg	
Total Carbohydrate 145g	
Dietary Fiber 22g	
Sugars 40g	
Protein 90g	

Calories Per Gram:
Fat 9 – Carbohydrate 4 – Protein 4

Breakfast
Cinnamon Cottage Cheese and Banana
with Shredded Wheat

Serves 2

1 cup	**low-fat cottage cheese**
1 medium	**banana, peeled and sliced**
1/2 teaspoon	**cinnamon**
1/4 teaspoon	**vanilla extract**
1 teaspoon	**Splenda®**
1 cup	**Shredded Wheat, spoon size**

Directions

1. Place all ingredients except Shredded Wheat into a small mixing bowl and mix well.

To serve, divide into 2 equal portions and top each with 1/2 cup Shredded Wheat. Serve immediately.

Nutrition Facts

Servings Per Meal: 2

Amount Per Serving

Calories 240 Calories from Fat 25

Total Fat 2.5g

Saturated Fat 1.5g

Trans Fat 0g

Cholesterol 10mg

Sodium 460mg

Total Carbohydrate 38g

Dietary Fiber 4g

Sugars 8g

Protein 19g

Calories Per Gram:
Fat 9 – Carbohydrate 4 – Protein 4

Lunch
Chicken Dijon Green Bean and Potato Salad

Serves 4

1 cup	canned potatoes, drained and chopped
1-1/2 cups	canned green beans, drained
1/2 cup	red onions, sliced thin
1 cup	tomatoes, chopped
1 medium	red bell pepper, diced
1-1/2 tablespoons	olive oil
3 tablespoons	white wine vinegar
1 tablespoon	Dijon mustard
2 tablespoons	fresh parsley, minced
1 pinch	salt and pepper, to taste
10 ounces	canned chicken, drained

Directions

1. Place all ingredients into a large bowl; mix well.

2. Chill and serve.

Nutrition Facts

Servings Per Meal: 4

Amount Per Serving

Calories 240   Calories from Fat 100

Total Fat 11g

Saturated Fat 2.5g

Trans Fat 0g

Cholesterol 35mg

Sodium 480mg

Total Carbohydrate 16g

Dietary Fiber 5g

Sugars 4g

Protein 21g

Calories Per Gram:
Fat 9 – Carbohydrate 4 – Protein 4

Dinner
Easy Scallop Bake

Serves 4

1 cup	brown rice, uncooked
3 cloves	garlic, chopped
2 cups	low sodium chicken broth
1 pound	scallops
1/4 cup	almonds, slivered
1/2 cup	carrots, diced
1/2 cup	celery, diced
1/2 cup	green bell pepper
1/2 cup	green onions, chopped
1 large	tomato, seeded and chopped
1/4 cup	fresh parsley, chopped

Nutrition Facts

Nutrition Facts

Servings Per Meal: 4

Amount Per Serving

Calories 360   Calories from Fat 60

Total Fat 7g

   Saturated Fat 1g

   Trans Fat 0g

Cholesterol 35mg

Sodium 260mg

Total Carbohydrate 48g

   Dietary Fiber 5g

   Sugars 4g

Protein 28g

Calories Per Gram:
Fat 9 – Carbohydrate 4 – Protein 4

Directions

1. Preheat oven to 350° F.

2. Combine brown rice, garlic, and chicken broth into a 9 x 13 inch baking dish.

3. Stir in scallops, almonds, and vegetables.

4. Cover baking pan with aluminum foil and place in preheated oven for 1 hour or until rice is done.

*Note: For crock pot cooking, place all ingredients into slow cooker and let cook for 6 to 8 hours on medium.

Daily Menu

Breakfast

- o Vanilla Whole Grain Pancakes with Sugar Free Maple Syrup

Mid Morning Snack

- o 125 Calorie Snack

Lunch

- o Quickie Albacore Tuna Salad w/Reduced Fat Whole Wheat Crackers

Mid Afternoon Snack

- o 100 Calorie Snack

Dinner

- o Hearty Turkey Lasagna Rolls

Evening Snack

- o 50 Calorie Snack

Nutrition Facts
Daily Menu
Amount Per Serving
Calories 1200 Calories from Fat 325
Total Fat 36g
Saturated Fat 8g
Trans Fat 0g
Cholesterol 188mg
Sodium 1615mg
Total Carbohydrate 138g
Dietary Fiber 24g
Sugars 29g
Protein 82g

Calories Per Gram:
Fat 9 – Carbohydrate 4 – Protein 4

Breakfast
Vanilla Whole Grain Pancakes
with Sugar Free Maple Syrup

Serves 8

1-3/4 cups	whole wheat pastry flour
1/2 cup	wheat germ
2 teaspoons	baking powder
1 tablespoon	granulated sugar
1-1/2 teaspoons	vanilla extract
1 large	egg
3 large	egg whites
2-1/2 cups	nonfat milk
1/2 cup	nonfat dry milk
1/4 cup	walnuts, chopped

Serve with:

1 cup	pancake syrup, sugar free
8 teaspoons	light tub margarine

Nutrition Facts

Servings Per Meal: 8

Amount Per Serving

Calories 260   Calories from Fat 70

Total Fat 8g

Saturated Fat 1g

Trans Fat 0g

Cholesterol 25mg

Sodium 310mg

Total Carbohydrate 38g

Dietary Fiber 5g

Sugars 8g

Protein 11g

Calories Per Gram:
Fat 9 – Carbohydrate 4 – Protein 4

Directions

1. In a medium bowl, add flour, wheat germ, baking powder, and sugar; mix well.

2. Add vanilla extract, egg, egg whites, nonfat milk, nonfat dry milk, and walnuts to dry mix; mix well.

3. Heat griddle over medium heat.

4. Spray griddle with nonstick cooking spray.

5. Using a 1/3 cup measuring cup to measure; pour the batter onto the griddle.

6. Turn pancake when bubbles come to the surface and the edges are slightly dry.

To serve, portion 2 pancakes, 1 teaspoon margarine, and 2 tablespoons sugar free syrup per serving.

Lunch
Quickie Albacore Tuna Salad
with Reduced Fat Whole Wheat Crackers

Serves 4

12 ounces	white albacore tuna* in water, drained
2 cups	romaine lettuce, chopped
1/2 cup	red onion, minced
1/4 cup	yellow bell pepper, chopped
1/4 cup	parsley, chopped
1/2 cup	tomatoes, chopped
1 clove	garlic, minced
1/2 teaspoon	black pepper
1 tablespoon	fresh dill, chopped
4 tablespoons	fresh lemon juice
2 tablespoons	extra virgin olive oil
16	reduced fat whole wheat crackers

Nutrition Facts
Servings Per Meal: 4

Amount Per Serving

Calories 250 Calories from Fat 80

Total Fat 10g

Saturated Fat 1g

Trans Fat 0g

Cholesterol 25mg

Sodium 390mg

Total Carbohydrate 18g

Dietary Fiber 3g

Sugars 2g

Protein 24g

Calories Per Gram:
Fat 9 – Carbohydrate 4 – Protein 4

Directions

1. In a large bowl, break albacore into bite sized pieces.

2. Add remaining ingredients, except crackers.

3. Gently toss to combine flavors.

4. Cover and refrigerate at least 4 hours before serving.

To serve, divide tuna salad into 4 equal portions and serve each with 4 reduced fat whole wheat crackers.

*Note: Tilapia and shrimp can also be substituted.

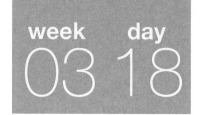

Dinner
Hearty Turkey Lasagna Rolls

Serves 6

1 pound	**ground turkey breast**
1 teaspoon	**Italian seasoning**
1 cup	**mushrooms, chopped**
1 medium	**onion, finely chopped**
1 small	**carrot, minced**
1 clove	**garlic, minced**
1/4 cup	**dry red wine**
1/8 teaspoon	**nutmeg**
1/2 cup	**part skim milk mozzarella cheese, shredded**
1/4 cup	**ricotta cheese, part skim**
1 large	**egg, lightly beaten**
12 ounces	**whole wheat lasagna noodles, cooked and drained**
16 ounces	**canned tomatoes, pureed**

Directions

1. Preheat oven to 350° F.
2. In a large non stick skillet, thoroughly brown ground turkey; drain fat.
3. Add Italian seasoning, mushrooms, onion, carrot and garlic; sauté until vegetables are tender.
4. Add wine, and nutmeg; cook until wine is almost evaporated.
5. Remove from heat; allow to cool 10 to 15 minutes.
6. In a medium bowl, thoroughly combine meat mixture, mozzarella cheese, ricotta cheese, and egg.
7. Pour half can of pureed tomato evenly in a 9 x 13 inch baking dish.
8. Evenly spread 1/3 cup meat filling over length of each lasagna noodle.
9. Carefully roll up noodle. Place seam side down in baking dish.
10. Repeat with remaining noodles.
11. Evenly spread remaining sauce over lasagna rolls.
12. Bake, covered, 40 minutes.

Breakfast

o Ricotta Raspberry Vanilla Whip with Graham Crackers

Mid Morning Snack

o 100 Calorie Snack

Lunch

o Asian Shrimp Pasta Salad with Plum

Mid Afternoon Snack

o 175 Calorie Snack

Dinner

o Turkey Apple Rice Stir-Fry

Evening Snack

o 75 Calorie Snack

Nutrition Facts	
Daily Menu	
Amount Per Serving	
Calories 1200 Calories from Fat 225	
Total Fat 25g	
Saturated Fat 7g	
Trans Fat 0g	
Cholesterol 255mg	
Sodium 1970mg	
Total Carbohydrate 160g	
Dietary Fiber 16g	
Sugars 58g	
Protein 83g	

Calories Per Gram:
Fat 9 – Carbohydrate 4 – Protein 4

Breakfast
Ricotta Raspberry Vanilla Whip
with Graham Crackers

Serves 1

1/3 cup	part skim ricotta cheese
1 cup	fresh raspberries
2 teaspoons	Splenda®
1/2 teaspoon	vanilla extract
4 squares	graham crackers

Directions

1. Place ricotta cheese, raspberries, Splenda®, and vanilla extract into small bowl and blend until creamy.

2. Remove mixture and chill until ready to serve.

To serve, spread mixture over graham crackers.

Nutrition Facts
Servings Per Meal: 1

Amount Per Serving

Calories 290   Calories from Fat 60

Total Fat 6 g

Saturated Fat 3g

Trans Fat 0g

Cholesterol 25mg

Sodium 350mg

Total Carbohydrate 54g

Dietary Fiber 1g

Sugars 11g

Protein 11g

Calories Per Gram:
Fat 9 – Carbohydrate 4 – Protein 4

Lunch
Asian Shrimp Pasta Salad
with Plum

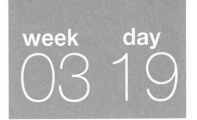
Serves 4

1 cup	whole wheat shell pasta, cooked
8 ounces	cooked shrimp, cut into chunks
2 cups	spinach leaves, stems removed and cut into strips
1/2 cup	fresh bean sprouts
1/2 small	red bell pepper, cut into thin strips
2	green onions, sliced

Dressing:

2 tablespoons	red wine vinegar
2 teaspoons	low sodium soy sauce
1 teaspoon	sesame oil
2 teaspoons	canola oil
2 teaspoons	teriyaki sauce
1 teaspoon	chili sauce
1 teaspoon	fresh ginger, grated
2 tablespoons	slivered almonds, toasted
8 large	plums, seeded and chopped

Nutrition Facts

Nutrition Facts

Servings Per Meal: 4

Amount Per Serving

Calories 230   Calories from Fat 60

Total Fat 7g

Saturated Fat 0.5g

Trans Fat 0g

Cholesterol 145mg

Sodium 560mg

Total Carbohydrate 28g

Dietary Fiber 4g

Sugars 14g

Protein 16g

Calories Per Gram:
Fat 9 – Carbohydrate 4 – Protein 4

Directions

1. Prepare pasta according to package directions; drain.

2. In large mixing bowl, combine pasta, shrimp, spinach, sprouts, pepper, and green onions.

3. In a small mixing bowl, mix together remaining ingredients except almonds; whisk well.

4. Toss dressing with pasta mixture and refrigerate until ready to serve.

To serve, divide shrimp salad into 4 equal portions, sprinkle almonds over top, and serve each portion with 1/2 cup chopped plum.

Dinner
Turkey Apple Rice Stir-Fry

Serves 6

1 tablespoon	butter
1/4 cup	carrots, cut into thin strips
1/4 cup	green onions, sliced
1-1/2 pounds	turkey breast cutlets, cut into thin strips
2 cups	apples, peeled, cored, and chopped
1 cup	brown rice, uncooked
2 tablespoons	seedless raisins
1 teaspoon	sesame seeds
1 small	red bell pepper, cut into thin strips
1 cup	frozen peas, thawed
1/2 teaspoon	salt
2 cups	low sodium chicken broth

Directions

1. Heat butter in large skillet over medium-high heat.

2. Cook and stir carrots 3 to 5 minutes until tender-crisp.

3. Add onions, turkey, and apples; cook 3 to 5 minutes.

4. Stir in rice, raisins, sesame seed, red bell pepper, peas, and salt.

5. Add chicken broth and bring to a boil; cover and let simmer for 30 minutes or until rice is tender.

Nutrition Facts
Servings Per Meal: 6

Amount Per Serving

Calories 320   Calories from Fat 35

Total Fat 4g

Saturated Fat 1.5g

Trans Fat 0g

Cholesterol 50mg

Sodium 340mg

Total Carbohydrate 37g

Dietary Fiber 4g

Sugars 9g

Protein 34g

Calories Per Gram:
Fat 9 – Carbohydrate 4 – Protein 4

Daily Menu

Breakfast

- o Banana Bran Muffins with Peanut Butter

Mid Morning Snack

- o 100 Calorie Snack

Lunch

- o Caribbean Chicken Salad

Mid Afternoon Snack

- o 150 Calorie Snack

Dinner

- o Beef Ratatouille

Evening Snack

- o 50 Calorie Snack

Nutrition Facts
Daily Menu
Amount Per Serving
Calories 1200 Calories from Fat 440
Total Fat 49g
Saturated Fat 14g
Trans Fat 0g
Cholesterol 195mg
Sodium 1550mg
Total Carbohydrate 112g
Dietary Fiber 18g
Sugars 48g
Protein 79g
Calories Per Gram: Fat 9 – Carbohydrate 4 – Protein 4

Breakfast

Banana Bran Muffins

with Peanut Butter

Serves 24*

6 cups	**Grape Nut Flakes**
5 cups	**whole wheat flour**
5 teaspoons	**baking soda**
3 cups	**Splenda®**
4 large	**eggs**
1 quart	**low-fat buttermilk**
1 teaspoon	**vanilla extract**
1 cup	**unsweetened applesauce**
6 large	**bananas, mashed**
1/2 tablespoon	**natural peanut butter per muffin**

Directions

1. Thoroughly mix all ingredients except peanut butter.

2. Store in fridge for up to one week.

3. Bake fresh as needed.

4. Fill muffin cups 2/3 full.

5. Bake at 400° F for 20 minutes.

One serving is 2 muffins and 1 tablespoon of peanut butter.

*Note: Recipe yields 48 muffins or 24 servings

Nutrition Facts	
Servings Per Meal: 24	
Amount Per Serving	
Calories 300	Calories from Fat 90
Total Fat 10g	
Saturated Fat 1.5g	
Trans Fat 0g	
Cholesterol 35mg	
Sodium 430mg	
Total Carbohydrate 44g	
Dietary Fiber 6g	
Sugars 10g	
Protein 11g	

Calories Per Gram:
Fat 9 – Carbohydrate 4 – Protein 4

Lunch
Caribbean Chicken Salad

Serves 4

12-1/2 ounces	canned chicken, drained
2 cups	mixed greens, chopped
1/4 cup	green bell pepper, chopped
8 ounces	crushed pineapple in water, drained
1/2 cup	grapes, cut in half
2 tablespoons	pimiento, sliced
1/2 cup	nonfat plain yogurt
1/4 cup	light mayonnaise
1-1/2 tablespoons	fresh lemon juice
1 teaspoon	curry powder
1/4 teaspoon	black pepper

Directions

1. Combine chicken, mixed greens, green pepper, pineapple, grapes, and pimiento.

2. In small bowl blend remaining ingredients.

3. Stir until well blended.

4. Pour over chicken mixture.

5. Toss lightly until well mixed; chill.

Nutrition Facts
Servings Per Meal: 4

Amount Per Serving

Calories 280   Calories from Fat 110

Total Fat 12g

Saturated Fat 2.5g

Trans Fat 0g

Cholesterol 50mg

Sodium 260mg

Total Carbohydrate 19g

Dietary Fiber 2g

Sugars 15g

Protein 24g

Calories Per Gram:
Fat 9 – Carbohydrate 4 – Protein 4

Dinner
Beef Ratatouille

Serves 4

1 teaspoon	olive oil
1 medium	onion, cut into wedges
3/4 pound	beef tenderloin, cut into thin strips
1 clove	garlic, minced
1 cup	eggplant, peeled and cut into 1 inch cubes
1 cup	zucchini, cut into 1" cubes
1 cup	green bell peppers, cut into 1" pieces
1 cup	canned, diced tomatoes
1/4 teaspoon	black pepper
1/2 teaspoon	dried basil
1/2 teaspoon	dried oregano

Directions

1. Heat oil in sauté pan.

2. Add onion, beef tenderloin and garlic; sauté for 5 minutes.

3. Add eggplant; sauté 2 minutes.

4. Add zucchini and peppers; sauté 5 minutes or until vegetables are still crisp and brightly colored.

5. Add remaining ingredients; simmer uncovered for 5 minutes.

Nutrition Facts
Servings Per Meal: 4

Amount Per Serving

Calories 310   Calories from Fat 170

Total Fat 19g

Saturated Fat 7g

Trans Fat 0g

Cholesterol 75mg

Sodium 135mg

Total Carbohydrate 10g

Dietary Fiber 4g

Sugars 5g

Protein 24g

Calories Per Gram:
Fat 9 – Carbohydrate 4 – Protein 4

Daily Menu

Breakfast
o Cheesy Spinach Cilantro Omelet with Whole Wheat Toast

Mid Morning Snack
o 100 Calorie Snack

Lunch
o Savory Seafood Soup with Oyster Crackers

Mid Afternoon Snack
o 150 Calorie Snack

Dinner
o Roasted Root Vegetables and Pork

Evening Snack
o 75 Calorie Snack

Nutrition Facts
Daily Menu

Amount Per Serving

Calories 1200 Calories from Fat 425

Total Fat 47g

Saturated Fat 12g

Trans Fat 0g

Cholesterol 254mg

Sodium 1885

Total Carbohydrate 100g

Dietary Fiber 17g

Sugars 33g

Protein 93g

Calories Per Gram:
Fat 9 – Carbohydrate 4 – Protein 4

Breakfast
Cheesy Spinach Cilantro Omelet
with Whole Wheat Toast

Serves 4

3/4 cup	frozen spinach, cooked and drained well
2 ounces	light cream cheese, diced
1 clove	garlic, minced
1 pinch	black pepper
1 tablespoon	cilantro, chopped
1/4 cup	Monterey jack cheese, shredded
1-1/2 cups	egg substitute
4 slices	whole wheat bread, toasted
4 teaspoons	light tub margarine

Directions

1. Preheat oven to 350° F.

2. Grease 4 individual baking dishes or ramekins with non-stick spray.

3. Combine all ingredients and divide between dishes.

4. Bake 20 minutes or until center is solid and puffy.

Serve each portion with 1 slice toast and 1 teaspoon margarine.

Nutrition Facts

Servings Per Meal: 4

Amount Per Serving

Calories 280 Calories from Fat 130

Total Fat 15g

   Saturated Fat 6g

   Trans Fat 0g

Cholesterol 20mg

Sodium 500mg

Total Carbohydrate 16g

   Dietary Fiber 3g

   Sugars 2g

Protein 22g

Calories Per Gram:
Fat 9 – Carbohydrate 4 – Protein 4

Lunch
Savory Seafood Soup
with Oyster Crackers

Serves 6

2 tablespoons	canola oil
1 large	onion, thinly sliced
1 cup	green onion, chopped
3 cloves	garlic, finely chopped
1/2 cup	fresh parsley, chopped
1 large	green bell pepper, seeded and diced
2-1/2 cups	low sodium tomato sauce
1/2 cup	dry white wine
1 cup	low sodium chicken broth
1/4 teaspoon	thyme, chopped fine
1/4 teaspoon	rosemary, chopped fine
1/4 teaspoon	fresh ground black pepper
1 each	bay leaf
1 pound	shrimp, peeled and deveined
1/2 pound	scallops
1-1/2 cups	oyster crackers

Nutrition Facts

Nutrition Facts
Servings Per Meal: 6

Amount Per Serving

Calories 300   Calories from Fat 70

Total Fat 8g

Saturated Fat 1g

Trans Fat 0g

Cholesterol 125mg

Sodium 320mg

Total Carbohydrate 24g

Dietary Fiber 3g

Sugars 7g

Protein 26g

Calories Per Gram:
Fat 9 – Carbohydrate 4 – Protein 4

Directions

1. Heat canola oil over medium high heat and add onions and garlic; cook, covered, over low heat until soft.

2. Add parsley, bell pepper, tomato sauce, wine, chicken broth, thyme, rosemary, black pepper, and bay leaf; cover and simmer for 1 hour.

3. Add shrimp and scallops, bring to a simmer; cover for 8-10 minutes or until seafood is cooked.

4. Remove bay leaf before serving.

To serve, divide into 6 equal portions and serve each with 1/4 cup oyster crackers.

Dinner
Roasted Root Vegetables and Pork

Serves 6

2 medium	onions, thinly sliced
3/4 pound	potatoes, peeled and cut into 2" pieces
1/2 pound	carrots, cut into 2" pieces
6 cloves	garlic, crushed
3 tablespoons	olive oil
1 teaspoon	dried dill
1 pound	lean pork loin, cut into 2" pieces
2 teaspoons	lime juice
2 teaspoons	chili powder
1/2 teaspoon	salt
1/4 teaspoon	black pepper

Nutrition Facts

Nutrition Facts

Servings Per Meal: 6

Amount Per Serving

Calories 290   Calories from Fat 130

Total Fat 14g

Saturated Fat 3.5g

Trans Fat 0g

Cholesterol 60mg

Sodium 270mg

Total Carbohydrate 15g

Dietary Fiber 3g

Sugars 4g

Protein 24g

Calories Per Gram:
Fat 9 – Carbohydrate 4 – Protein 4

Directions

1. Preheat oven to 400° F.

2. Toss cut vegetables, oil, dill, pork, lime juice, chili powder, pepper, and salt in a bowl.

3. Transfer vegetables and pork to the baking sheet and roast in a 400° F oven for about 45 minutes, or until pork reaches 170° F.

4. During the last 30 minutes of roasting, toss every 10 minutes to ensure burning does not occur on any one side.

Note: Use different types of herbs or spices in place of dill weed (such as rosemary, basil, or gram macula for an Indian flavor).

Daily Menu

Breakfast

o Pear Spiced Oatmeal Bread Pudding

Mid Morning Snack

o 125 Calorie Snack

Lunch

o White Bean and Chicken Chili

Mid Afternoon Snack

o 125 Calorie Snack

Dinner

o Angel Hair with Sesame Shrimp Sauce

Evening Snack

o 100 Calorie Snack

Nutrition Facts	
Daily Menu	
Amount Per Serving	
Calories 1200	Calories from Fat 225
Total Fat 25g	
Saturated Fat 4g	
Trans Fat 0g	
Cholesterol 210mg	
Sodium 2195mg	
Total Carbohydrate 158g	
Dietary Fiber 32g	
Sugars 55g	
Protein 87g	

Calories Per Gram:
Fat 9 – Carbohydrate 4 – Protein 4

Breakfast
Pear Spiced Oatmeal Bread Pudding

Serves 6

6 slices	**day-old whole wheat bread, cubed**
3/4 cup	**quick cooking oats, uncooked**
1 cup	**egg substitute, beaten**
2 cups	**canned pears, in juice, drained and diced**
2-1/2 cups	**nonfat milk**
1/2 cup	**Splenda®**
1 tablespoon	**vanilla**
1 tablespoon	**apple pie spice**

Directions

1. Preheat oven to 350° F.

2. In a large bowl place cubed day-old bread.

3. Add oatmeal, egg substitute, pears, milk, Splenda®, vanilla, and apple pie spice to bread cubes; mix well.

4. Place mixture in an 8 x 8 inch baking dish which has been sprayed with non-stick cooking spray.

5. Bake until pudding has risen high and medium brown, about 30 minutes. It will rise like a soufflé and fall as it cools.

Note: The sugar from this recipe is naturally occurring from the fruit and dairy.

Nutrition Facts
Servings Per Meal: 6

Amount Per Serving

Calories 230   Calories from Fat 30

Total Fat 3g

Saturated Fat 0g

Trans Fat 0g

Cholesterol 0mg

Sodium 280mg

Total Carbohydrate 39g

Dietary Fiber 4g

Sugars 15g

Protein 13g

Calories Per Gram:
Fat 9 – Carbohydrate 4 – Protein 4

Lunch
White Bean and Chicken Chili

Serves 6

1 tablespoon	canola oil
1 large	onion, chopped
4 cloves	garlic, finely chopped
1 large	red bell pepper, chopped
2 each	jalapenos, seeded and chopped
1 tablespoon	ground cumin
2 teaspoons	ground coriander
1/2 teaspoon	cayenne pepper
1/4 teaspoon	black pepper
2 cups	canned white beans, drained and rinsed
28 ounces	canned no salt added tomatoes, broken up
14 ounces	tomato sauce
5-1/2 ounces	unsalted tomato paste
3/4 pound	boneless skinless chicken breast, cooked and cut into pieces
1 cup	frozen green beans
2 tablespoons	fresh cilantro, chopped
2 tablespoons	fresh lime juice

Nutrition Facts

Servings Per Meal: 6

Amount Per Serving

Calories 290   Calories from Fat 45

Total Fat 5g

  Saturated Fat 1g

  Trans Fat 0g

Cholesterol 50mg

Sodium 500mg

Total Carbohydrate 37g

  Dietary Fiber 12g

  Sugars 13g

Protein 27g

Calories Per Gram:
  Fat 9 – Carbohydrate 4 – Protein 4

Directions

1. In a large saucepan or skillet, heat oil over medium heat.

2. Sauté onion, garlic, pepper, and dried seasonings over low heat for about 20 minutes.

3. Add beans, tomatoes, tomato sauce, and tomato paste.

4. Simmer gently for 20 minutes.

5. Stir in cooked chicken and green beans and cook until heated through.

6. Before serving, add fresh cilantro and lime juice; stir gently.

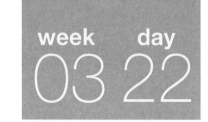

Dinner
Angel Hair with Sesame Shrimp Sauce

Serves 6

8 ounces	whole wheat angel hair pasta, uncooked
1 pound	asparagus tips, trimmed and cut into 1-inch pieces
2 teaspoons	canola oil
5 cloves	garlic, chopped
1 cup	mushrooms, sliced
1/4 cup	low sodium soy sauce
1 tablespoon	sesame oil
1 tablespoon	brown sugar
2 tablespoons	chutney
2 tablespoons	toasted sesame seeds
1/2 cup	green onions, chopped
1/2 cup	white vinegar
1 pound	shrimp, raw

Nutrition Facts

Nutrition Facts

Servings Per Meal: 6

Amount Per Serving

Calories 310   Calories from Fat 60

Total Fat 7g

Saturated Fat 1g

Trans Fat 0g

Cholesterol 115mg

Sodium 520mg

Total Carbohydrate 39g

Dietary Fiber 7g

Sugars 7g

Protein 24g

Calories Per Gram:
Fat 9 – Carbohydrate 4 – Protein 4

Directions

1. Prepare pasta according to package directions; two minutes before pasta is done, add asparagus tips.

2. When pasta and asparagus are done, drain.

3. Place oil, garlic, and mushrooms in a 2-quart saucepan.

4. Sauté for 3 to 4 minutes.

5. Add soy sauce, sesame oil, brown sugar, chutney, toasted sesame seeds, green onions, and vinegar; simmer for 3 to 5 minutes.

6. Add shrimp to the sauce; cook for 5 to 8 minutes.

7. Toss shrimp and sauce with pasta and asparagus.

Daily Nutritional Average

Nutrition Facts
Weekly Daily Average

Amount Per Serving

Calories 1200 Calories from Fat 315

Total Fat 35g

Saturated Fat 10g

Trans Fat 0g

Cholesterol 230mg

Sodium 2065mg

Total Carbohydrate 135g

Dietary Fiber 20g

Sugars 46g

Protein 91g

Calories Per Gram:
Fat 9 – Carbohydrate 4 – Protein 4

Week 4 Recipes

Day 23   Alpine Vegetable Quiche
Lemon Blueberry Turkey Salad
Just For the Halibut Stir-Fry

Day 24   Canadian Bacon Cheese Toast
Slow Cooked Chicken 'n Olives
Spaghetti and Spinach Tomato Feta Pesto Bake

Day 25   Cinnamon Ricotta Peach Spread and Rice Cakes
Turkey Caesar Pocket
Rum Marinate Beef Tenderloin and Cilantro Roasted Potatoes

Day 26   Guiltless Shrimp and Brie Scrambled Eggs
Pork Arroz Con Queso
Pan Seared Tilapia on Linguini with Tomato Cream Sauce

Day 27   Fluffy Vanilla Cinnamon French Toast with Bananas and Almonds
Tossed Tuna Garden Salad
Chicken Carbinade

Day 28   Toasty Cheese Sandwich with Herbed Mayonnaise
Well Thymed Turkey Meatloaf
Garlic Parmesan Sauce Over Corkscrew Pasta and Scallops

Day 29   Cheery Cherry Brunch Pie
Sooner Chopped Pork Salad
Homemade Chicken Pot Pie Lasagna

Day 30   Mexican Scramble Breakfast Pita*
Hungarian Goulash Soup
Sierra Primavera with Orange Roughy

*Extra day in week 4 to accommodate 30 full days of recipes.

Week 4 Shopping List

Baking Products
baking mix, reduced fat — 1 cup

Bread Products
bread, rye — 1 slice
bread, whole wheat — 7 slices
English muffins, whole wheat — 2
pita bread, whole wheat — 8 small

Canned Beans
black beans, low sodium — 8 ounces
pinto beans — 16 ounces

Canned Fruits
cherries, unsweetened tart — 16 ounces
peaches, in juice — 1 cup

Canned Seafood & Meat
albacore, in water — 6 ounces

Canned Vegetables
whole tomatoes, low sodium — 16 ounces

Cereals
wheat bran — 1 cup

Condiments
chili sauce — 1 teaspoon
chutney — 2 tablespoons

Dairy Products
Brie cheese — 2 ounces
butter — 1 tablespoon
cheddar cheese, low-fat, shredded — 1 cup
cottage cheese, low-fat — 2-1/2 cups
egg whites — 2 large
eggs — 10 large
feta cheese, reduced fat — 8 ounces
heavy cream — 2 tablespoons
margarine, light tub — 3 tablespoons
milk, 1% — 1-1/2 cups
milk, 2% — 1/3 cup
milk, nonfat — 5 cups

Monterey jack cheese, reduced fat — 1 cup shredded
Monterey jack cheese with jalapeno — 1/2 cup shredded
mozzarella cheese, part skim — 1-1/2 cups shredded
parmesan cheese, fresh — 1 cup shredded
ricotta cheese, part skim — 16 ounces
sour cream, light — 4 teaspoons
Swiss cheese, low-fat — 4 ounces shredded
yogurt, light lemon — 6 ounces

Deli Lunchmeat
Canadian bacon — 1 slice
turkey breast, low sodium — 1 pound

Dried Beans & Rice
brown rice, dry — 1-1/2 cups

Fresh Seafood & Fish
halibut steaks — 1 pound
orange Roughy — 1 pound
scallops, fresh — 1-1/2 pounds
bay shrimp, fresh — 3/4 cup
tilapia — 1 pound

Frozen Foods
egg substitute — 2-3/4 cups
butternut squash — 4 cups
peas — 1 cup
spinach, chopped — 10 ounces

Jams & Jellies
100% fruit spread — 4 tablespoons

Meat & Poultry
beef chuck, lean — 2 pounds
beef tenderloin — 1-1/2 pounds
chicken breasts, boneless skinless — 4 pounds
pork tenderloin — 1 pound
turkey breast, ground — 2 pounds
turkey sausage, fresh — 8 ounces

Mexican Food Products
green chilies, canned — 1 4 ounce can
refried beans, fat-free, canned — 1/2 cup

Nuts & Seeds
almonds   1 tablespoon

Pasta
couscous, dry   1 cup
pasta, whole wheat corkscrew   8 ounces
pasta, whole wheat, dry   4 ounces
pasta, whole wheat linguini   4 ounces
pasta, whole wheat, lasagna   12 pieces
protein plus spaghetti, dry   1 pound

Pickles & Olives
black olives, sliced   1/4 cup
olives, green or black   1/2 cup

Produce
avocado   1 medium
banana   1 medium
basil leaves, fresh   1 tablespoon
Bibb lettuce   2 cups
blackberries   3 cups
blueberries   2 cups
broccoli flowerets   4 cups
carrots   2 large
celery   1 stalk
cherry tomatoes   2 1/2 cups
chives, fresh   1 teaspoon
cilantro, fresh   2 tablespoons
cucumber   1 large
garlic   15 cloves
ginger, fresh   1 tablespoon
honeydew melon   2 small
iceberg lettuce   1/2 cup
Italian parsley, fresh   1/2 cup
kiwi fruits   2
lemon juice   4 teaspoons
lemon zest   1 teaspoon
lime juice   2 tablespoons
mangos   3 large

mixed salad greens   1 cup
mushrooms   2 pounds
onions, green   2 bunches
onion, red   1 medium
onions, yellow   10 large
parsley, fresh   1/4 cup
pepper, green bell   1 small
pepper, red bell   1 medium
potatoes   5 pounds
romaine lettuce   2 cups
shallot   1
tomatoes   8 large
tomatoes, plum   7 large
watermelon   1 cup
zucchini   3 large

Refrigerated Pasta
pesto sauce, reduced fat   2 tablespoons

Salad Dressings
Caesar, reduced calorie   2 tablespoons
Italian, reduced calorie   1/4 cup

Soups
beef broth, low sodium   1 cup
chicken broth, low sodium   2 cups

Spirits for Cooking
beer   3/4 cup
dry sherry   1/2 cup
nonalcoholic beer   12 ounces
rum   1/2 cup
white wine   1 cup

Tomato Sauces
tomato paste   1 tablespoon
tomato sauce, low sodium   8 ounces

Breakfast

o Alpine Vegetable Quiche with Honeydew Melon

Mid Morning Snack

o 150 Calorie Snack

Lunch

o Lemon Blueberry Turkey Salad with Graham Crackers

Mid Afternoon Snack

o 150 Calorie Snack

Dinner

o Just For the Halibut Stir-Fry and Baked Potato

Evening Snack

o 50 Calorie Snack

Nutrition Facts
Daily Menu
Amount Per Serving
Calories 1200 Calories from Fat 305
Total Fat 34g
Saturated Fat 7g
Trans Fat 0g
Cholesterol 310mg
Sodium 1695mg
Total Carbohydrate 130g
Dietary Fiber 16g
Sugars 58g
Protein 94g

Calories Per Gram:
Fat 9 – Carbohydrate 4 – Protein 4

Breakfast
Alpine Vegetable Quiche
with Honeydew Melon

Serves 6

1/2 cup	onion, diced
1/2 cup	green bell pepper, diced
1 teaspoon	olive oil
1 cup	mushrooms, sliced
1/2 cup	low-fat Swiss cheese, shredded
1-1/2 cups	low-fat cottage cheese
1/2 teaspoon	black pepper
4 large	eggs
1/3 cup	2% low-fat milk
1 tablespoon	parsley, chopped or dried
6 cups	honeydew melon, chopped

Directions

1. Preheat oven to 400° F.
2. Coat a 9-inch round baking dish with nonstick cooking spray.
3. Sauté onions and peppers in olive oil in nonstick skillet for about 5 minutes.
4. Add mushrooms; continue cooking for about 3 more minutes.
5. Combine Swiss cheese, cottage cheese, and black pepper in a medium bowl; set aside.
6. Beat eggs for about two minutes.
7. Add milk, and parsley; continue to beat for another minute or so.
8. Place half the cheese mixture in the prepared baking dish.
9. Add the cooked pepper-onion-mushroom mixture; layer with remaining cheese mixture.
10. Pour egg mixture on top.
11. Bake for about 35 minutes or until a knife inserted in center comes out clean.
12. Let rest for 5 to 10 minutes before serving.

To serve, divide quiche into 6 equal portions and serve each with 1 cup honeydew melon.

Nutrition Facts

Servings Per Meal: 6

Amount Per Serving

Calories 200   Calories from Fat 50

Total Fat 6g

 Saturated Fat 2.5g

 Trans Fat 0g

Cholesterol 150mg

Sodium 340mg

Total Carbohydrate 21g

 Dietary Fiber 2g

 Sugars 16g

Protein 17g

Calories Per Gram:
Fat 9 – Carbohydrate 4 – Protein 4

Lunch
Lemon Blueberry Turkey Salad
with Graham Crackers

Serves 4

2 cups	fresh blueberries, divided
6 ounces	light lemon yogurt
3 tablespoons	light mayonnaise
12 ounces	low sodium turkey breast*, cooked and cubed
1/2 cup	green onions, chopped
3/4 cup	cucumber, peeled and chopped
1/2 cup	red bell pepper, diced
4 squares	graham crackers

Directions

1. Reserve a few blueberries for garnish.

2. In a medium bowl, combine yogurt, and mayonnaise.

3. Add remaining blueberries, the turkey, green onions, cucumbers, and bell pepper; mix gently.

4. Cover and refrigerate to let flavors blend, at least 30 minutes.

5. Place mix over endive or other greens garnished with reserved blueberries and lemon slices, if desired.

To serve, divide salad into 4 equal portions and serve each with 1 graham cracker square.

*Note: Fish or seafood can also be used.

Nutrition Facts

Servings Per Meal: 4

Amount Per Serving

Calories 260   Calories from Fat 50

Total Fat 5g

   Saturated Fat 1g

   Trans Fat 0g

Cholesterol 75mg

Sodium 200mg

Total Carbohydrate 24g

   Dietary Fiber 3g

   Sugars 14g

Protein 29g

Calories Per Gram:
Fat 9 – Carbohydrate 4 – Protein 4

Dinner
Just for the Halibut Stir-Fry
and Baked Potato

Serves 4

1 pound	halibut steak, cut into 4 ounce steaks
1 medium	tomato, diced
1/2 cup	fresh mushrooms, sliced
1/2 cup	onions, sliced
1/2 cup	celery, diced
1 tablespoon	lemon juice
2 teaspoons	canola oil
1/4 teaspoon	thyme, ground
1/8 teaspoon	salt
1 pinch	black pepper
4 medium	baked potatoes
8 teaspoons	light tub margarine
4 teaspoons	light sour cream

Directions

1. Preheat oven to 375° F.

2. To cook potato, rinse and wrap with foil and place in oven for 45 minutes or until fork tender.

3. Sprinkle halibut with salt and pepper; place in shallow baking dish.

4. In a large preheated non stick sauté pan add tomato, mushrooms, onions, celery, lemon juice, oil, thyme, salt and pepper; sauté until tender.

5. Spoon over halibut.

6. Place covered halibut into oven and bake for 10 minutes or until halibut flakes when tested with a fork.

Serve each potato with 2 teaspoons margarine, 1 teaspoon light sour cream, and halibut stir-fry.

Nutrition Facts
Servings Per Meal: 4

Amount Per Serving

Calories 390   Calories from Fat 120

Total Fat 13g

  Saturated Fat 2g

  Trans Fat 0g

Cholesterol 40mg

Sodium 270mg

Total Carbohydrate 39g

  Dietary Fiber 3g

  Sugars 6g

Protein 28g

Calories Per Gram:
Fat 9 – Carbohydrate 4 – Protein 4

Breakfast
o Canadian Bacon Cheese Toast with Watermelon

Mid Morning Snack
o 125 Calorie Snack

Lunch
o Slow Cooked Chicken 'n Olives with Mango

Mid Afternoon Snack
o 100 Calorie Snack

Dinner
o Spaghetti and Spinach Tomato Feta Pesto Bake

Evening Snack
o 75 Calorie Snack

Nutrition Facts
Daily Menu
Amount Per Serving
Calories 1200 Calories from Fat 250
Total Fat 28g
Saturated Fat 8g
Trans Fat 0g
Cholesterol 135mg
Sodium 2270mg
Total Carbohydrate 158g
Dietary Fiber 21g
Sugars 61g
Protein 83g
Calories Per Gram: Fat 9 – Carbohydrate 4 – Protein 4

Breakfast
Canadian Bacon Cheese Toast
with Watermelon

Serves 1

1 slice	**whole wheat bread, toasted**
1 teaspoon	**light tub margarine**
1 slice	**Canadian bacon**
2 tablespoons	**low-fat cheddar cheese, shredded**
1 cup	**watermelon, cubed**

Directions

1. Spread toasted whole wheat bread with margarine.

2. Top with Canadian bacon and cheese.

3. Place in oven 5 inches from broiler and broil for 2 minutes. While broiling watch carefully to keep from burning toast.

Serve with watermelon on the side.

Nutrition Facts
Servings Per Meal: 1

Amount Per Serving

Calories 220   Calories from Fat 70

Total Fat 8g

Saturated Fat 2g

Trans Fat 0g

Cholesterol 15mg

Sodium 660mg

Total Carbohydrate 26g

Dietary Fiber 3g

Sugars 11g

Protein 13g

Calories Per Gram:
Fat 9 – Carbohydrate 4 – Protein 4

Lunch
Slow Cooked Chicken 'n Olives
with Mango

Serves 6

1-1/2 pounds	boneless skinless chicken breast, cut into small pieces
1/2 teaspoon	black pepper
1 clove	garlic, minced
1 large	onion, chopped
1 cup	carrots, sliced
2 each	bay leaves
3/4 cup	beer
8 ounces	low sodium tomato sauce
1/2 cup	green olives
1-1/2 cups	brown rice, cooked
6 cups	mango, peeled and chopped

Nutrition Facts
Servings Per Meal: 6

Amount Per Serving

Calories 360   Calories from Fat 40

Total Fat 4.5g

Saturated Fat 0.5g

Trans Fat 0g

Cholesterol 65mg

Sodium 360mg

Total Carbohydrate 49g

Dietary Fiber 5g

Sugars 28g

Protein 29g

Calories Per Gram:
Fat 9 – Carbohydrate 4 – Protein 4

Directions

1. Rinse chicken pieces and pat dry; lightly season with pepper.

2. Combine all ingredients except rice in crock pot; stir well.

3. Cover and cook on low setting for 7 to 9 hours. Remove bay leaf before serving.

4. Serve over cooked rice.

To serve, divide into 6 equal portions and serve each with 1 cup chopped mango.

Dinner
Spaghetti and Spinach Tomato Feta Pesto Bake

Serves 8

1 pound	protein plus spaghetti, uncooked
10 ounces	frozen chopped spinach, thawed and drained
1/2 cup	parmesan cheese, grated
2 tablespoons	water
8 ounces	reduced fat feta cheese, crumbled
2 tablespoons	reduced fat refrigerated pesto sauce
6 large	plum tomatoes cut into 2" pieces

Directions

1. Preheat oven to 350° F.

2. Prepare pasta according to package directions; drain.

3. Toss cooked warm pasta with thawed spinach, parmesan cheese, water, feta cheese, plum tomatoes, and pesto sauce.

4. Spray a 9 X 13 inch baking dish with nonstick cooking spray.

5. Put pasta mixture into pan, cover with aluminum foil, and bake for 20 minutes.

Nutrition Facts
Servings Per Meal: 8

Amount Per Serving

Calories 320   Calories from Fat 70

Total Fat 8g

  Saturated Fat 3g

  Trans Fat 0g

Cholesterol 15mg

Sodium 530mg

Total Carbohydrate 44g

  Dietary Fiber 6g

  Sugars 4g

Protein 20g

Calories Per Gram:
Fat 9 – Carbohydrate 4 – Protein 4

Breakfast
- o Cinnamon Ricotta Peach Spread and Rice Cakes

Mid Morning Snack
- o 100 Calorie Snack

Lunch
- o Turkey Caesar Pocket

Mid Afternoon Snack
- o 100 Calorie Snack

Dinner
- o Rum Marinated Beef Tenderloin and Cilantro Roasted Potatoes

Evening Snack
- o 100 Calorie Snack

Nutrition Facts
Daily Menu
Amount Per Serving
Calories 1200 Calories from Fat 415
Total Fat 46g
Saturated Fat 15g
Trans Fat 0g
Cholesterol 195mg
Sodium 1670mg
Total Carbohydrate 112g
Dietary Fiber 17g
Sugars 36g
Protein 83g

Calories Per Gram:
Fat 9 – Carbohydrate 4 – Protein 4

Breakfast
Cinnamon Ricotta Peach Spread and Rice Cakes

Serves 1

1/3 cup	part skim ricotta cheese
1/2 teaspoon	cinnamon
1 packet	Splenda®
1/2 cup	diced peaches, canned, in juice or water, drained
2 large	brown rice cakes

Directions

1. In a small bowl, combine ricotta cheese, peaches, cinnamon, and Splenda®; mix well.

2. Spread mixture over rice cakes and serve.

Note: 2 large rice cakes equals 4 mini rice cakes.

Nutrition Facts
Servings Per Meal: 1

Amount Per Serving

Calories 250   Calories from Fat 60

Total Fat 7g

Saturated Fat 4g

Trans Fat 0g

Cholesterol 25mg

Sodium 115mg

Total Carbohydrate 37g

Dietary Fiber 2g

Sugars 13g

Protein 10g

Calories Per Gram:
Fat 9 – Carbohydrate 4 – Protein 4

Lunch
Turkey Caesar Pocket

Serves 4

2 cups	romaine lettuce, shredded
2 tablespoons	parmesan cheese, grated
4	green onions, chopped
2 tablespoons	vinegar-based reduced calorie Caesar salad dressing
4 small	whole wheat pita bread
8 ounces	low sodium turkey slices
1 medium	avocado, peeled and sliced
1 pinch	black pepper, to taste

Directions

1. In medium bowl, combine lettuce, cheese, green onion, and salad dressing.

2. Stuff each half of pita with 1/2 cup mixture and top each with 2 slices turkey and avocado; pepper to taste.

Nutrition Facts

Servings Per Meal: 4

Amount Per Serving

Calories 240   Calories from Fat 90

Total Fat 10g

  Saturated Fat 2g

  Trans Fat 0g

Cholesterol 30mg

Sodium 560mg

Total Carbohydrate 23g

  Dietary Fiber 6g

  Sugars 2g

Protein 19g

Calories Per Gram:
  Fat 9 – Carbohydrate 4 – Protein 4

Dinner

Rum Marinated Beef Tenderloin and Cilantro Roasted Potatoes

Serves 6

1/2 cup	rum
1 tablespoon	olive oil
1 tablespoon	chili powder
2 cloves	garlic, chopped
1 teaspoon	ground oregano
1/4 teaspoon	hot pepper sauce
1-1/2 pounds	beef tenderloin, cut into 6- 4 ounce pieces

Rum Marinated Beef Tenderloin Directions

1. Mix rum with next 5 ingredients for marinade.

2. Marinate steaks in the refrigerator 30 minutes to 2 hours. Discard marinade once used.

3. Grill steaks until medium rare.

Recipe continued on next page...

Nutrition Facts

Servings Per Meal: 6

Amount Per Serving

Calories 390   Calories from Fat 190

Total Fat 22g

  Saturated Fat 8g

  Trans Fat 0g

Cholesterol 100mg

Sodium 270mg

Total Carbohydrate 13g

  Dietary Fiber 2g

  Sugars 2g

Protein 32g

Calories Per Gram:
Fat 9 – Carbohydrate 4 – Protein 4

Dinner (continued)
Rum Marinated Beef Tenderloin and Cilantro Roasted Potatoes

Cilantro Roasted Potatoes:

1/2 tablespoon	olive oil
1/2 tablespoon	chili powder
1 teaspoon	garlic, chopped
1/2 teaspoon	salt
1/4 teaspoon	black pepper
3/4 pound	potatoes, unpeeled and cut into wedges
1/2 medium	onion, cut into thick wedges
1-1/2 cups	cherry tomatoes, halved
2 tablespoons	cilantro, chopped
2 tablespoons	lime juice

Cilantro Roasted Potatoes Directions

1. Preheat oven to 425° F.

2. On lightly-oiled nonstick baking sheet, combine all seasoning ingredients.

3. Add potatoes and onion; toss to coat evenly.

4. Bake 25 minutes.

5. Add tomatoes; bake an additional 7 to 10 minutes or until potatoes are tender.

6. Transfer vegetables to large bowl; add cilantro.

7. Sprinkle with lime juice; toss lightly.

Daily Menu

Breakfast

o Guiltless Shrimp and Brie Scrambled Eggs with Whole Wheat English Muffin

Mid Morning Snack

o 100 Calorie Snack

Lunch

o Pork Arroz Con Queso

Mid Afternoon Snack

o 100 Calorie Snack

Dinner

o Pan Seared Tilapia on Linguini with Tomato Cream Sauce

Evening Snack

o 100 Calorie Snack

Nutrition Facts
Daily Menu

Amount Per Serving

Calories 1200 Calories from Fat 315

Total Fat 35g

Saturated Fat 13g

Trans Fat 0g

Cholesterol 255mg

Sodium 1925mg

Total Carbohydrate 123g

Dietary Fiber 18g

Sugars 35g

Protein 98g

Calories Per Gram:
Fat 9 – Carbohydrate 4 – Protein 4

Breakfast
Guiltless Shrimp and Brie Scrambled Eggs
with Whole Wheat English Muffin

Serves 4

1-1/4 cups	egg substitute
1/4 cup	nonfat milk
2 ounces	Brie cheese
1 pinch	salt, pepper, and cayenne pepper, to taste
1 teaspoon	chives, minced
3/4 cup	bay shrimp, cooked
2 each	whole wheat English muffin, cut in half
4 tablespoons	100% fruit spread

Directions

1. Mix egg substitute and milk together.

2. Cut Brie into small pieces; add with seasonings and chives to egg mixture.

3. Melt butter in 8" frying pan over medium heat.

4. Place egg mixture in pan with shrimp.

5. Stir until well cooked and fluffy.

To serve, divide eggs into 4 equal portions and serve each with 1/2 toasted English muffin and 1 tablespoon fruit spread.

Nutrition Facts
Servings Per Meal: 4

Amount Per Serving

Calories 270   Calories from Fat 70

Total Fat 8g

Saturated Fat 3g

Trans Fat 0g

Cholesterol 100mg

Sodium 480mg

Total Carbohydrate 24g

Dietary Fiber 2g

Sugars 12g

Protein 27g

Calories Per Gram:
Fat 9 – Carbohydrate 4 – Protein 4

Lunch
Pork Arroz Con Queso

Serves 6

6 ounces	pork tenderloin, cut into small cubes
3/4 cup	brown rice, uncooked
16 ounces	canned whole tomatoes, low sodium, mashed
16 ounces	canned pinto beans, drained and rinsed
3 cloves	garlic, minced
1 large	onion, finely chopped
1 cup	low-fat cottage cheese
4 ounces	canned green chili peppers, drained
1 cup	reduced fat Monterey jack cheese, shredded

Directions

1. Mix thoroughly all ingredients except cheese.

2. Pour mixture into crock-pot sprayed with nonstick cooking spray.

3. Cover and cook on low setting for 6 to 9 hours.

4. Garnish with cheese before serving.

Nutrition Facts

Servings Per Meal: 6

Amount Per Serving

Calories 310   Calories from Fat 70

Total Fat 8g

Saturated Fat 3.5g

Trans Fat 0g

Cholesterol 40mg

Sodium 560mg

Total Carbohydrate 37g

Dietary Fiber 7g

Sugars 4g

Protein 25g

Calories Per Gram:
Fat 9 – Carbohydrate 4 – Protein 4

Dinner

Pan Seared Tilapia on Linguine with Tomato Cream Sauce

Serves 4

1 cup	dry white wine
1/4 cup	shallots, minced
2 tablespoons	fresh lime juice
1 tablespoon	fresh ginger, peeled and grated
2 tablespoons	heavy cream
1 tablespoon	butter, cut into small pieces
2/3 cup	plum tomatoes, seeded and chopped
2 tablespoons	fresh cilantro, chopped
1/4 teaspoon	salt
1/8 teaspoon	black pepper
2 cups	whole wheat linguini, cooked
1 coat	cooking spray
1 pound	tilapia, cut into 4 equal pieces

Nutrition Facts

Servings Per Meal: 4

Amount Per Serving

Calories 310   Calories from Fat 70

Total Fat 8g

Saturated Fat 4g

Trans Fat 0g

Cholesterol 75mg

Sodium 230mg

Total Carbohydrate 24g

Dietary Fiber 2g

Sugars 1g

Protein 27g

Calories Per Gram:
Fat 9 – Carbohydrate 4 – Protein 4

Directions

1. Combine first 4 ingredients in a medium skillet; bring to a boil.
2. Cook until reduced to 1/2 cup (about 5 minutes).
3. Add cream; cook over medium heat 1 minute.
4. Add butter, stirring until butter melts.
5. Stir in tomato, cilantro, salt, and pepper.
6. Add linguine; toss well. Cover and keep warm.
7. Heat a large nonstick skillet coated with cooking spray over medium-high heat.
8. Arrange tilapia in pan; cook 3 minutes on each side or until done.
9. Add tilapia to pasta mixture; toss gently to combine.
10. Garnish with cilantro, if desired.

Breakfast
- o Fluffy Vanilla Cinnamon French Toast with Bananas and Almonds

Mid Morning Snack
- o 150 Calorie Snack

Lunch
- o Tossed Tuna Garden Salad

Mid Afternoon Snack
- o 175 Calorie Snack

Dinner
- o Chicken Carbinade with Couscous and Broccoli

Evening Snack
- o 125 Calorie Snack

Nutrition Facts
Daily Menu

Amount Per Serving

Calories 1200 Calories from Fat 335

Total Fat 37g

Saturated Fat 6g

Trans Fat 0g

Cholesterol 145mg

Sodium 2290mg

Total Carbohydrate 117g

Dietary Fiber 20g

Sugars 45g

Protein 97g

Calories Per Gram:
Fat 9 – Carbohydrate 4 – Protein 4

Breakfast
Fluffy Vanilla Cinnamon French Toast with Bananas and Almonds

Serves 4

1-1/2 cups	egg substitute
1 cup	nonfat milk
1/2 teaspoon	vanilla extract
1 teaspoon	cinnamon
6 slices	whole wheat bread
1 coat	nonstick pan spray
1 cup	banana, sliced
1 tablespoon	almonds, slivered

Directions

1. Whisk together egg substitute, milk, vanilla, and cinnamon until light and frothy.

2. Dip bread slices in egg mixture and place on greased (use non-stick cooking spray) baking pan.

3. Pour any leftover mixture over bread slices; cover and refrigerate overnight.

4. Next day, sauté bread on non-stick griddle until light brown and crispy.

5. Top with bananas and almonds.

*Note: Sugar-free syrup can be used if desired. 1 serving is 1 1/2 slices of bread.

Nutrition Facts
Servings Per Meal: 4

Amount Per Serving

Calories 250   Calories from Fat 50

Total Fat 6g

Saturated Fat 1g

Trans Fat 0g

Cholesterol 0mg

Sodium 390mg

Total Carbohydrate 30g

Dietary Fiber 4g

Sugars 11g

Protein 20g

Calories Per Gram:
Fat 9 – Carbohydrate 4 – Protein 4

Lunch
Tossed Tuna Garden Salad

Serves 2

6 ounces	albacore tuna, canned in water; drain and flaked
1/4 small	red onion, sliced thin
1 medium	tomato, chopped
1/2 medium	red bell pepper, chopped
1 cup	assorted salad greens
1 tablespoon	fresh basil, chopped
1/2 cup	carrot, shredded
4 teaspoons	canola oil
2 teaspoons	Dijon mustard
1/2 teaspoon	balsamic vinegar

Directions

1. In a large bowl, combine the albacore, onion, tomato, red pepper, salad greens, basil, and carrots; mix well.

2. In a separate bowl, mix the canola oil, mustard, and vinegar.

3. Add the dressing mixture and tuna to the salad greens and combine thoroughly.

4. Portion evenly onto chilled serving plates.

Nutrition Facts
Servings Per Meal: 2

Amount Per Serving

Calories 230   Calories from Fat 90

Total Fat 10g

  Saturated Fat 1g

  Trans Fat 0g

Cholesterol 25mg

Sodium 380mg

Total Carbohydrate 10g

  Dietary Fiber 3g

  Sugars 6g

Protein 23g

Calories Per Gram:
  Fat 9 – Carbohydrate 4 – Protein 4

Dinner
Chicken Carbinade
with Couscous and Broccoli

Serves 8

1-1/2 pounds	boneless skinless chicken breast, cut into 1" cubes
1-1/4 teaspoons	salt
1 teaspoon	black pepper
4 tablespoons	canola oil
4 large	onions, sliced
1 tablespoon	tomato paste
2 cloves	garlic, chopped
3 tablespoons	all-purpose flour
1 cup	low sodium beef broth
1 cup	low sodium chicken broth
12 ounces	nonalcoholic beer
2 each	bay leaves
1 teaspoon	thyme
1 tablespoon	cider vinegar
2 cups	couscous, cooked
4 cups	broccoli florets, steamed

Nutrition Facts
Servings Per Meal: 8

Amount Per Serving

Calories 270   Calories from Fat 80

Total Fat 9g

  Saturated Fat 1g

  Trans Fat 0g

Cholesterol 50g

Sodium 480mg

Total Carbohydrate 22g

  Dietary Fiber 3g

  Sugars 4g

Protein 24g

Calories Per Gram:
Fat 9 – Carbohydrate 4 – Protein 4

Directions

1. Preheat oven to 350° F.
2. Pat chicken cubes dry; salt and pepper cubes.
3. In large sauté pan over medium high heat add 2 tablespoons canola oil.
4. When oil is heated sauté chicken in 3 batches; don't touch for 2 minutes to get a good sear. Set aside.
5. Add remaining oil over medium low heat.
6. Add onion and tomato paste; keep on medium low for 5 minutes and stir.
7. Turn heat up to medium and cook until golden brown.
8. Add garlic to onions.
9. Add flour; cook for 3 minutes.
10. Add beef broth, chicken broth, beer, bay leaf, thyme, and vinegar.
11. Bring to a full simmer.
12. Add chicken; place in oven for 2 to 2.5 hours with lid cracked.

To serve, divide into 8 equal portions and serve each with 1/4 cup couscous and 1/2 cup steamed broccoli.

Breakfast

o Toasty Cheese Sandwich with Herbed Mayonnaise and Peaches

Mid Morning Snack

o 125 Calorie Snack

Lunch

o Well Thymed Turkey Meatloaf with Winter Squash

Mid Afternoon Snack

o 125 Calorie Snack

Dinner

o Garlic Parmesan Sauce Over Corkscrew Pasta and Scallops with Blackberries

Evening Snack

o 50 Calorie Snack

Nutrition Facts		
Daily Menu		
Amount Per Serving		
Calories 1200 Calories from Fat 290		
Total Fat 32g		
Saturated Fat 8g		
Trans Fat 0g		
Cholesterol 150mg		
Sodium 2215mg		
Total Carbohydrate 145g		
Dietary Fiber 27g		
Sugars 52g		
Protein 86g		

Calories Per Gram:
Fat 9 – Carbohydrate 4 – Protein 4

Breakfast
Toasty Cheese Sandwich with Herbed Mayonnaise

and Peaches

Serves 1

Herbed Mayonnaise

1/2 cup	light mayonnaise
1/4 teaspoon	onion powder
1/4 teaspoon	chili powder
1/8 teaspoon	dried basil
1/2 teaspoon	fresh lemon juice
1 slice	rye bread, toasted
1 ounce	cheddar cheese, low-fat
1-1/2 teaspoons	light herbed mayonnaise
1 half	peach, canned in juice

Nutrition Facts	
Servings Per Meal: 1	
Amount Per Serving	
Calories 240	Calories from Fat 50
Total Fat 6g	
Saturated Fat 2g	
Trans Fat 0g	
Cholesterol 10mg	
Sodium 450mg	
Total Carbohydrate 39g	
Dietary Fiber 4g	
Sugars 22g	
Protein 11g	

Calories Per Gram:
Fat 9 – Carbohydrate 4 – Protein 4

Directions

1. Place all herbed mayo ingredients into a small bowl and mix well.

2. Place in refrigerator for 1 hour.

3. Spread toasted rye bread with 1-1/2 teaspoons herbed mayo.

4. Place cheddar cheese on top of mayo and fold in half.

Serve peach half on the side.

*Note: Reserve extra mayo in airtight container and use for other recipes.

Lunch
Well Thymed Turkey Meatloaf
with Butternut Squash

Serves 8

1 medium	onion, diced small
1 tablespoon	olive oil
3 cloves	garlic, minced
2 teaspoons	dried thyme
1 teaspoon	dried sage
1/2 teaspoon	black pepper
2 pounds	lean ground turkey
1 cup	wheat bran
4 tablespoons	ketchup
1 tablespoon	Worcestershire sauce
1/2 cup	Italian parsley, chopped fine
2 large	egg whites, beaten
4 cups	butternut squash, cooked according to package directions

Directions

1. Preheat oven to 350° F.
2. Sauté onions and garlic in olive oil until translucent but not brown.
3. Add the herbs; sauté for 2 minutes.
4. Place the turkey in a bowl and add the bran, ketchup, Worcestershire sauce, parsley, and egg whites; mix well.
5. Stir in the cooled onion mixture.
6. Spray a 9 x 5 x 3 inch loaf pan with nonstick cooking spray and place the turkey mixture into the pan.
7. Bake the loaf approximately 1 hour 20 minutes to an internal temperature of 160° F.

To serve, divide the meatloaf into 8 equal portions and serve each with 1/2 cup of butternut squash.

Note: Can also be made into meatballs and baked in the oven.

Nutrition Facts
Servings Per Meal: 8

Amount Per Serving

Calories 270   Calories from Fat 100

Total Fat 11g

    Saturated Fat 3g

    Trans Fat 0g

Cholesterol 90mg

Sodium 510mg

Total Carbohydrate 21g

    Dietary Fiber 7g

    Sugars 8g

Protein 24g

Calories Per Gram:
  Fat 9 – Carbohydrate 4 – Protein 4

Dinner

Garlic Parmesan Sauce Over Cork Screw Pasta and Scallops

with Blackberries

Serves 6

8 ounces	whole wheat pasta (cork screw shaped), uncooked
1 tablespoon	garlic, minced
1 tablespoon	olive oil
1 pound	fresh mushrooms, sliced
1 cup	low sodium chicken broth
2 tablespoons	cornstarch
1/2 teaspoon	salt
1/4 teaspoon	ground black pepper
2 cups	zucchini, cut in 1 inch pieces
1-1/2 pounds	scallops
1 cup	cherry tomatoes, cut in half
1/4 cup	parmesan cheese, shredded
3 cups	blackberries

Nutrition Facts

Servings Per Meal: 6

Amount Per Serving

Calories 350 Calories from Fat 50

Total Fat 6g

Saturated Fat 1g

Trans Fat 0g

Cholesterol 40mg

Sodium 450mg

Total Carbohydrate 46g

Dietary Fiber 8g

Sugars 6g

Protein 24g

Calories Per Gram:
Fat 9 – Carbohydrate 4 – Protein 4

Directions

1. Cook pasta according to manufacturer's directions; drain and put in a large serving bowl.

2. Preheat a sauté pan and add olive oil and garlic.

3. When the garlic begins to sizzle, add mushrooms and sauté until soft.

4. In a cup combine chicken broth, cornstarch, salt, and black pepper until smooth; stir into mushrooms.

5. Bring to a simmer; cook for 4 minutes.

6. Add zucchini, scallops, and cherry tomatoes; simmer for an additional 5 minutes.

7. Stir in parmesan cheese; pour over reserved pasta; toss gently.

To serve divide into 6 equal portions and serve each with 1/2 cup blackberries.

Daily Menu

Breakfast
- o Cheery Cherry Brunch Pie

Mid Morning Snack
- o 125 Calorie Snack

Lunch
- o Sooner Chopped Pork Salad

Mid Afternoon Snack
- o 150 Calorie Snack

Dinner
- o Homemade Chicken Pot Pie Lasagna

Evening Snack
- o 50 Calorie Snack

Nutrition Facts	
Daily Menu	
Amount Per Serving	
Calories 1200	Calories from Fat 345
Total Fat 38g	
Saturated Fat 14g	
Trans Fat 0g	
Cholesterol 310mg	
Sodium 2285mg	
Total Carbohydrate 120g	
Dietary Fiber 20g	
Sugars 42g	
Protein 95g	

Calories Per Gram:
Fat 9 – Carbohydrate 4 – Protein 4

Breakfast
Cheery Cherry Brunch Pie

Serves 6

1/2 pound	turkey sausage
1 16 ounce can	unsweetened tart cherries*, drained and coarsely chopped
1/2 cup	low-fat cheddar cheese, shredded
1 cup	reduced fat baking mix
1 teaspoon	dried basil
1/8 teaspoon	black pepper
4 large	eggs
1-1/2 cups	1% milk

Directions

1. Preheat oven to 400° F.

2. In a large skillet, cook sausage until brown, breaking into small pieces as it cooks; drain off fat.

3. Remove from heat.

4. Add cherries; mix well.

5. Spoon sausage mixture into a 10-inch deep-dish pie plate; top with cheese.

6. In a medium mixing bowl, combine baking mix, basil, and pepper.

7. Add eggs and milk; beat until smooth. Pour over cheese.

8. Bake 35 to 40 minutes, or until a knife inserted in center comes out clean.

9. Let cool 5 minutes.

Serving Ideas: Serve with a mixed green salad.

* Note: 1-1/2 cups frozen unsweetened tart cherries can be substituted for canned cherries. Partially thaw cherries, then coarsely chop, and drain before adding to sausage.

Week 4

Lunch
Sooner Chopped Pork Salad

Serves 4

2 cups	Bibb lettuce, torn into bite size pieces
1/2 pound	lean pork tenderloin, cooked and shredded
8 ounces	low sodium canned black beans, drained
8 ounces	fresh mushrooms, quartered
2 large	tomatoes, chopped
1/2 cup	Monterey jack cheese with jalapeno, shredded
1/4 cup	pitted black olives, sliced
1/4 cup	low calorie Italian salad dressing
1/2 teaspoon	chili powder

Directions

1. Place lettuce in a large serving bowl.

2. In a medium bowl, combine pork, beans, mushrooms, tomatoes, cheese and olives; spoon over lettuce.

3. Combine dressing and chili powder; pour over salad and toss gently.

Nutrition Facts

Servings Per Meal: 4

Amount Per Serving

Calories 260   Calories from Fat 110

Total Fat 12g

Saturated Fat 5g

Trans Fat 0g

Cholesterol 55mg

Sodium 540mg

Total Carbohydrate 16g

Dietary Fiber 5g

Sugars 4g

Protein 24g

Calories Per Gram:
Fat 9 – Carbohydrate 4 – Protein 4

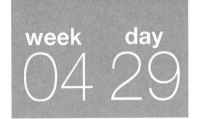
Dinner
Homemade Chicken Pot Pie Lasagna

Serves 10

12 pieces	**whole wheat lasagna, uncooked**
1 pound	**boneless skinless chicken breast, diced**
3 cups	**fresh mushrooms, sliced**
1 cup	**carrots, thinly sliced**
1/2 cup	**green onions, sliced**
1 cup	**frozen green peas, thawed and well drained**

Directions

1. Prepare pasta according to package directions.

2. Spray a large sauté pan with cooking spray; place over medium-high heat until hot.

3. Add chicken and sauté 4 minutes or until cooked through.

4. Drain well and set aside.

5. Recoat sauté pan with cooking spray and place over medium-high heat until hot.

6. Add mushrooms, carrots, green onions, and peas; sauté 6 minutes.

7. Set aside.

Recipe Continued on Next Page...

Nutrition Facts

Servings Per Meal: 10

Amount Per Serving	
Calories 360	Calories from Fat 80
Total Fat 9g	
Saturated Fat 4.5g	
Trans Fat 0g	
Cholesterol 50mg	
Sodium 350mg	
Total Carbohydrate 37g	
Dietary Fiber 6g	
Sugars 7g	
Protein 31g	

Calories Per Gram:
Fat 9 – Carbohydrate 4 – Protein 4

Dinner (continued)
Homemade Chicken Pot Pie Lasagna

Sauce:

1/2 cup	all-purpose flour
3-1/2 cups	nonfat milk
1/2 cup	dry sherry
1 teaspoon	ground thyme
1/2 teaspoon	salt
1/4 teaspoon	cayenne pepper
15 ounces	part skim ricotta cheese
1-1/2 cups	part skim mozzarella cheese, grated and divided
1/2 cup	reduced fat Swiss cheese, shredded

Sauce Directions

1. Preheat oven to 350° F.
2. Place flour in a medium saucepan.
3. Gradually add milk, stirring with a wire whisk until blended; stir in sherry.
4. Bring to a boil over medium heat; cook for 5 minutes or until thickened, stirring constantly.
5. Stir in thyme, salt, and cayenne pepper.
6. Reserve one cup of sauce and set aside.
7. In a bowl, combine ricotta cheese, 1 cup mozzarella, and Swiss cheese.
8. Spread 1 cup of the sauce over the bottom of a 13 x 9 x 2 inch pan.
9. Arrange 4 pieces of the lasagna (3 lengthwise, 1 widthwise) over the sauce.
9. Top with half of ricotta cheese mixture, half of chicken mixture, and half of remaining sauce mixture.
11. Repeat layers, ending with 4 pieces of lasagna.
12. Spread reserved 1 cup of sauce over the last complete layer of lasagna, being sure to cover the lasagna completely.
13. Cover lasagna with foil and bake 1 hour.
14. Uncover lasagna, sprinkle remaining 1/2 cup mozzarella cheese on top; bake an additional 5 minutes uncovered.
15. Re-cover and let stand 15 minutes before serving.

Daily Menu

Breakfast
o Mexican Scramble Breakfast Pita with Kiwi

Mid Morning Snack
o 125 Calorie Snack

Lunch
o Hungarian Goulash Soup

Mid Afternoon Snack
o 150 Calorie Snack

Dinner
o Sierra Primavera with Orange Roughy

Evening Snack
o 100 Calorie Snack

Nutrition Facts	
Daily Menu	
Amount Per Serving	
Calories 1200	Calories from Fat 290
Total Fat 32g	
Saturated Fat 8g	
Trans Fat 0g	
Cholesterol 350mg	
Sodium 2165mg	
Total Carbohydrate 136g	
Dietary Fiber 24g	
Sugars 39g	
Protein 93g	

Calories Per Gram:
Fat 9 – Carbohydrate 4 – Protein 4

Breakfast
Mexican Scramble Breakfast Pita
with Kiwi

Serves 2

2 large	eggs
1/4 teaspoon	black pepper
2 small	whole wheat pitas, warmed
1/2 cup	nonfat refried beans, warmed
1/4 cup	cooked diced potatoes, warmed
1/2 cup	shredded iceberg lettuce
1 large sprig	cilantro, chopped or sprig, for garnish
2 tablespoons	salsa
2 each	kiwi fruit, peeled and sliced

Directions

1. Scramble eggs with pepper.

2. Cook over medium heat until thoroughly cooked.

3. Fill warmed pita halves with warmed refried beans.

4. Top with warmed potatoes and shredded lettuce.

5. Add scrambled eggs, salsa, and garnish with cilantro.

Serve 1 kiwi on the side per portion.

Nutrition Facts
Servings Per Meal: 2

Amount Per Serving

Calories 260   Calories from Fat 45

Total Fat 5g

Saturated Fat 1.5g

Trans Fat 0g

Cholesterol 180mg

Sodium 620mg

Total Carbohydrate 41g

Dietary Fiber 8g

Sugars 9g

Protein 14g

Calories Per Gram:
Fat 9 – Carbohydrate 4 – Protein 4

Lunch
Hungarian Goulash Soup

Serves 8

2 medium	onions, peeled and chopped
2 large	cloves garlic, crushed
2 tablespoons	canola oil
2 tablespoons	paprika
2 pounds	lean beef chuck, cut into 1/2" cubes
2 large	tomatoes, peeled and chopped
2 teaspoons	caraway seeds
1-1/2 teaspoons	dried marjoram
1 teaspoon	lemon zest, minced
8 cups	water
1/2 teaspoon	black pepper
3 medium	potatoes, peeled and cubed

Nutrition Facts

Nutrition Facts

Servings Per Meal: 8

Amount Per Serving

Calories 270   Calories from Fat 80

Total Fat 9g

Saturated Fat 2g

Trans Fat 0g

Cholesterol 50mg

Sodium 90mg

Total Carbohydrate 19g

Dietary Fiber 3g

Sugars 3g

Protein 27g

Calories Per Gram:
Fat 9 – Carbohydrate 4 – Protein 4

Directions

1. Sauté onions and garlic in heated oil in a large sauté pan until tender.

2. Stir in paprika; cook 1 minute.

3. Brown beef cubes, several at a time, on all sides.

4. Add tomatoes, caraway seeds, marjoram, lemon zest, water, and pepper.

5. Bring to a boil. Lower heat and cook slowly, covered, 45 minutes.

6. Add potatoes and continue to cook about 20 minutes longer, until potatoes are tender.

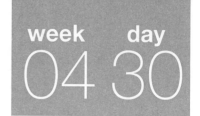

Dinner
Sierra Primavera with Orange Roughy

Serves 4

4 ounces	whole wheat pasta, uncooked
1 tablespoon	olive oil
1/2 teaspoon	salt
1 clove	garlic, minced
1/2 medium	red onion, chopped
2 cups	zucchini, chopped
1 pound	orange roughy
2 cups	fresh tomatoes, chopped
1/4 teaspoon	red pepper flakes
1/4 cup	nonfat milk
1/4 cup	parmesan cheese, grated
2 tablespoons	fresh parsley, chopped

Nutrition Facts

Servings Per Meal: *4*

Amount Per Serving

Calories 290 Calories from Fat 60

Total Fat 7g

Saturated Fat 1.5g

Trans Fat 0g

Cholesterol 75mg

Sodium 520mg

Total Carbohydrate 30g

Dietary Fiber 4g

Sugars 5g

Protein 29g

Calories Per Gram:
Fat 9 – Carbohydrate 4 – Protein 4

Directions

1. Prepare pasta according to package directions; drain.

2. Heat the oil in a large skillet.

3. Add the garlic, red onion, and zucchini and cook over medium-high heat until the garlic and onion are golden.

4. Reduce heat to medium and add the orange roughy, tomato, red pepper flakes, and nonfat milk; let simmer for 10 minutes.

5. Stir in cheese.

6. Add the pasta and parsley then mix thoroughly.

Smart Snacking

Smart snacking as the name implies is a very important contributor to weight loss. You may recall Chef Dave's first two goals he set out in his thoughts, Before You Begin. The first goal is to take ownership of what you eat. This is just as true for your main meals as it is for snacks. If you do not have a plan, then the most you can hope for is a plan to fail. With a small amount of advanced planning, you can make sure to have a snack ready for your prescribed snack time.

This goes hand in hand with Chef Dave's second key to success of eating 6 times per day. I know this does not seem intuitive; however, it's vital to weight loss and weight maintenance. In order for our metabolisms to function correctly and therefore burn instead of store fat, we have to provide the fuel necessary to do so. Snacking is critical to this mind set.

Another great point about smart snacking is that it plays well into the goal of watching portion sizes. Once we begin to understand what a portion is and how many calories it equates to, then we can become more informed consumers of calories.

Smart snacking also enforces the mind set of maintaining a daily caloric budget. Let's face it, humans as consumers of calories are not very in tune with what and how much to eat given the variety and accessibility to what is available. Certainly, from a weight loss and weight maintenance perspective, we have to maintain a caloric budget proportional to our individual resting metabolic rate combined with our output.

The snack lists allow you to customize your daily menu plans. You pick and choose the foods you wish to eat in between your regular mealtimes. The snack lists are put into four calorie levels: 25, 50, 75, and 100 calories. The lists are in 25 calorie blocks so you can mix and match foods from any of the list to equal the recommended calories per snack on your daily menu. Let's take a look at the 50 calorie snack list.

All the foods in the 50 calorie list average 50 calories for the serving size listed. The other nutrient levels within the list will vary depending upon the food. For example: Fruit is going to have more fiber and vitamin C than bread. Cottage cheese will have more protein than popcorn. If you choose a variety of foods from the lists, you will be eating a wider range of nutrients.

Now let's plan our snacks for Day 1.

Classic Egg and Cheese Breakfast Sandwich with Fresh Orange

6 oz. light yogurt (100 calorie list)

OR

1/4 cup low-fat cottage cheese (50 calorie list) with

1 cup cantaloupe cubes (50 calorie list)

Hurry Curry Pork Salad with Reduced Fat Whole Wheat Crackers

2 oz. low sodium deli turkey lunchmeat (50 calories) wrapped around

1 piece part skim string cheese (75 calories)

OR

1 oz. low-fat soy crisp crackers (100 calorie list) with

1/4 cup salsa (25 calorie list)

Chicken Cacciatore with Green Beans and Penne Pasta

1/2 cup unsweetened applesauce (50 calories) with

2 1/2 square graham crackers (50 calories)

OR

4 cups 94% fat-free microwave popcorn (2 cups = 50 calories)

Smart Snacking Tips

Smart snacking is NOT hit and miss eating; grabbing what is handy, or running to the vending machine. Here are tips and strategies you can use to make the most of snack time:

Don't skip meals. You will be tempted to eat more than you planned because you are hungry.

Eat meals and snacks at set times. Having a structured eating schedule will make it easier for you to manage your weight.

Stick to the serving sizes listed. Snacking does not mean "grazing" for an extended period of time on a buffet of foods.

Beware of eating triggers, those things that lead you down the road of overeating. Triggers can include certain foods, the time of day, locations, and the people around you.

Use the snack lists to make good choices and be sure to add them to your shopping list so you have them available.

Minimize access to foods that are hard for you to control.

If you are hungry, choose foods that are higher in fiber and water or are protein based.

Fruits and vegetables can help you feel fuller for less calories, plus they are packed with lots of "good for you" nutrients.

Eating tuna salad with crackers will be more filling than eating crackers alone. Check the lists for your serving sizes.

The best place to eat a snack is at the table. Eating in the car or in front of the computer or TV is usually mindless eating and leads to overeating.

Planning + Practice = Success

25 Calorie Food Snack List

Food	Amount	
American cheese, nonfat	1	slice
Broccoli, florets, fresh	1	cup
Carrots, baby	8	medium
Cauliflower, florets, fresh	1	cup
Cheddar cheese, low-fat, grated	2	tablespoons
Cheese, parmesan, grated	1	tablespoon
Cherries, fresh	1/4	cup
Cucumber, peeled	1	medium
Gelatin, sugar free	1	cup
Green beans, canned	1/2	cup
Green bell pepper, fresh	1	small
Mayonnaise, light	1 1/2	teaspoons
Peanut butter, natural, creamy	1	teaspoon
Red bell pepper, fresh	1	small
Salsa	1/4	cup
Shrimp, cooked	4	large
Summer squash, all types, fresh	1	small
Tomatoes, fresh	3/4	medium

50 Calorie Food Snack List

Food	Amount	
Almonds	7	nuts
Apple, fresh	1	small
Applesauce, unsweetened	1/2	cup
Apricots, fresh	2	each
Apricots, halves canned in juice	1/2	cup
Banana, medium	1/2	each
Beans, non-fat refried, canned	1/4	cup
Beef jerky	1/2	ounce
Blackberries, fresh	3/4	cup
Blueberries, fresh	3/4	cup
Bread, 100% whole wheat, reduced calorie	1	slice
Cantaloupe, fresh, cubes	1	cup
Chicken noodle soup, canned, prepared w/water	1/2	cup
Chickpeas	1/4	cup
Cottage cheese, 1% fat	1/4	cup
Deli turkey, low sodium	2	ounces
Fruit salad, canned in juice	1/2	cup

50 Calorie Food Snack List (cont.)

Food	Amount	
Graham crackers, 2 1/2" square	2	squares
Grapes, seedless, fresh	20	grapes
Honeydew melon, fresh, diced	1	cup
Hummus	2	tablespoons
Kiwi, fresh	1	medium
Mandarin oranges, canned in juice	3/4	cup
Mango, fresh, slices	1/2	cup
Melba toast, rye	3	pieces
Milk, nonfat	1/2	cup
Nectarine, fresh	1	medium
Orange, fresh	1	medium
Peach, fresh	1	medium
Peaches, halves, canned in juice	1/2	cup
Plum, fresh	1	medium
Popcorn, air popped	2	cups
Popcorn, microwave, 94% fat-free	2	cups
Raspberries, fresh	1	cup
Ricotta cheese, low-fat	1/4	cup
Saltine crackers	4	pieces
Soybeans, edamame	1/4	cup
Strawberries, fresh, sliced	1	cup
String cheese, reduced fat	1	piece
Vegetable soup, canned, prepared with water	1/2	cup
Watermelon, fresh, diced	1	cup
Whole wheat crackers, reduced fat	3	crackers

75 Calorie Food Snack List

Food	Amount	
Alpine Vegetable Quiche (pg. 110)	1/2	serving
Apples, fresh	1	medium
Asian Shrimp Pasta Salad (pg. 91)	1/2	serving
Avocado, fresh	1/4	each
Bread, rye	1	slice
Cereal, bran flakes	1/2	cup
Cereal, shredded wheat	1	large biscuit
Cheese, American	1	slice
English muffin, whole wheat	1/2	each
Herb Baked Eggs (pg. 10)	1/2	serving
Minestrone soup, canned	1	cup
Sausage and Cheddar Frittata (pg. 30)	1/2	serving
String cheese, part skim	1	piece
Tasty Tomato, Basil, and Cheese Frittata (pg. 53)	1/2	serving
Tofu, baked and flavored	2	ounces

100 Calorie Food Snack List

Food	Amount	
Almonds	14	nuts
Banana Bran Muffin (94)	1	muffin
Beans, no fat refried, canned	1/2	cup
Beef jerky	1	ounce
Black beans, low sodium, canned	1/2	cup
Canadian bacon	2	ounces
Egg, hard cooked	1	egg
Oatmeal, plain cooked	3/4	cup
Pears, fresh	1	medium
Ricotta cheese, low-fat	1/2	cup
Soy crisps, snack chips, low-fat	1	ounce
Soy nuts, roasted, and salted	1/4	cup
Swiss cheese, reduced fat	1	ounce
Three bean salad, canned	1/2	cup
Tomato soup, ready to serve	3/4	cup
Tuna fish, packed in water	3	ounces
Well Thymed Turkey Meatloaf (132)	1/2	serving
Yogurt, light, no sugar added	6	ounces

Glossary

Asiago Cheese: A cow's milk cheese made in northern Italy. Mild nutty flavor when young, more pronounced with age.

Brie Cheese: Made from cow's milk, this soft, creamy cheese has a delicate, slightly nutty flavor. The white rind is also edible.

Brown Rice: Whole rice grain with only the very outer husk removed. The bran coating is left on, giving the rice a tan color and nutlike flavor. Brown rice is higher in fiber and more nutritious than white rice.

Butternut Squash: A large, pear-shaped squash with a smooth yellow brown skin and orange flesh with a sweet flavor.

Chutney: From the Hindi chatni, it is a condiment made from fruit, vinegar, sugar and spices; its texture can range from smooth to chunky and its flavor from mild to hot.

Cilantro: The dark green lacy leaves of the cilantro plant; used as an herb, they have a sharp, tangy fresh flavor and aroma and are used fresh in Mexican, South American and Asian cuisines; also known as Chinese parsley.

Couscous: Small, spherical bits of semolina dough that are rolled, dampened and coated with finer wheat flour; a staple of the North African diet.

Curry Powder: An American or European blend of spices associated with Indian cuisines, the flavor and color vary depending on the exact blend; typical ingredients include black pepper, cinnamon, cloves, coriander, cumin, ginger, mace and turmeric, with cardamom, tamarind, fennel seeds, fenugreek, and/or chili powder is sometimes added.

Dry Mustard: Dry mustard is ground mustard seeds. These are used to make the mustard you are used to putting on your hot dog by mixing the dry mustard or mustard flour as it is sometimes know with water or sometimes beer. You can find dry mustard in the spice section of your local grocery store.

Feta Cheese:	A salty, soft Greek cheese made from ewe's milk and pickled in brine it has a white color, crumbly texture, and salty, sour, tangy flavor. A soft, white, flaky American feta-style cheese made from cow's milk and stored in brine.
Kalamata Olives:	A dark purple, fruity Greek olive.
Leek:	Has a thick, cylindrical white stalk with a slightly bulbous root end and dark green leaves. The tender, white stalk has a flavor that is sweeter and stronger than a scallion but milder than an onion.
Lemon Zest:	The thin, brightly colored outer part of the rind of citrus fruits. It contains volatile oils, used as a flavoring.
Low-fat:	A food containing 3 grams of fat or less per serving.
Low Sodium:	A food containing 140 milligrams or less per serving.
Light:	FDA term used to define food that has 33 percent fewer calories, 50 percent less fat, or 50 percent less sodium than the regularly used food.
Marsala Wine:	An Italian, dessert wine, served as an after dinner drink. Marsala is available in dry and sweet.
Nonfat:	Lacking fat solids or having the fat content removed.
Pimientos:	Large red, sweet pepper. Pimientos are usually found diced in cans and jars and are added to dishes to enhance the color and flavor.
Soba Noodles:	Japanese noodles containing buckwheat flour.
Summer Squash:	There are many varieties of this gourd including zucchini, yellow straight neck, yellow crookneck, and patty pan. All summer squash are similar in taste and texture.
Wheat Germ:	The embryo or seedling plant within the grain; containing concentrated Vitamin E, minerals, and protein.
Wondra® Quick-Mixing Flour:	Quick-Mixing Wondra® dissolves instantly, even in cold liquids. Patented agglomeration process turns this all-purpose flour into a quick mix wonder.

Cooking Resources

Dry Cooking Methods

Sauté	To cook food in a preheated pan or griddle with a minimum amount of fat
Rotisserie	To cook food in dry heat while food is rotating
Grilling	To cook food from heat below
Broiling	To cook food from heat above
Roasting	To cook food in dry heat with the aid of fat

Moist Cooking Methods

Deep Frying	To cook food in preheated fat or oil totally immersed
Pan Frying	To cook food in preheated fat or oil partially immersed
Stewing	To cook small pieces of food at below simmering point with liquid
Braising	To cook in a closed container with liquid in the oven or on top of the stove
Poaching	To cook food in a liquid at a temperature below boiling, i.e. ~ 160° F
Boiling	To cook in a liquid at 212° F

Cooking Equivalents

1/2 ounce (oz.)	1 tablespoon (tbsp.)
3 teaspoons (tsp.)	1 tbsp.
8 oz.	1 cup (c)
16 oz.	2 c = 1 pint (pt.)
32 oz.	2 pt. = 1 quart (qt.)
64 oz.	2 qt. = 1/2 gallon (gal.)
128 oz.	4 qt. = 1 gallon (gal.)
1 pound (#)	16 oz.

Liquid measure is different than dry measure so use correct measuring device to insure success in your recipe.

Cooking Temperature

Beef: 145° F for medium rare. Bacteria in beef are generally destroyed at this temperature. Ground beef, however, should be cooked at 160° F because of the larger surface area available for bacterial formation.

Chicken: 165° F for white meat, 185° F for dark meat. Salmonella is destroyed at 165° F.

Pork: 150° F for medium rare. Trichinosis is destroyed at 137° F.

Fish: 140° F opaque and flaky.

About the Author

Chef David Fouts received his Culinary Degree in 1994 from the Florida Culinary Institute in West Palm Beach, Florida. Soon thereafter, he was hired by the prestigious 5 Star Diamond Hotel "The Breakers" in West Palm Beach, where he worked for several years. Other professional appointments include Director of Food Services at Hippocrates Health Institute which is one of the premier vegan/vegetarian resorts in South Florida; Executive Chef for Omni Hotels; and Personal Chef for a family in Naples, Florida. He currently is the Corporate Chef for the International Metabolic Institute™ based in Reno, Nevada.

Over the last several years, Chef Dave has written, contributed and advised on several editorial boards for publications throughout the country. In 2003, he wrote his first book, **"Culinary Classics: Essentials of Cooking for the Gastric Bypass Patient."** The book was born out of his passion to help patients he works with on a daily basis and to help them overcome their challenges with food choices following weight loss surgery. It was this endeavor which led Chef Dave to co-author the first edition of **"Weight Loss Surgery for Dummies,"** as well as an invitation to the editorial board as a contributor for WLS Lifestyles magazine and writer/contributor for *Beyond Change*, *Bariatric Times* and several other health publications.

These days, you can find Chef Dave lecturing and performing cooking seminars across the country. He advises on food and product development for Fortune 500 companies. He was recently featured on the front cover of WLS Lifestyles Magazine in their quarterly issue. Besides his national speaking engagements, Chef Dave is proud to say he is kept very busy at home with his wife and two children. He is actively involved in his community and work, and enjoys leisure and travel time with his family.

About the Dietician

Vicki Bovee, M.S., R.D., is a registered dietitian/nutritionist with 25 years experience in weight loss and weight management. Her professional appointments include Clinical Dietitian, Western Bariatric Institute and faculty member of the University of Nevada School of Medicine. Vicki received her master's degree in nutrition from Montana State University and her Bachelor of Science degree in home economics from the University of Wisconsin-Stevens Point. She is a member of The American Dietetic Association and The Obesity Society.

Index

Poultry

Vegetarian

Other Books by 360 Publishing

Check for availability and ordering www.sasseguide.com

Outpatient Weight Loss Surgery
Safe and Successful Weight Loss with Modern Bariatric Surgery
Kent Sasse MD, MPH, FACS

Kent Sasse, MD, MPH, FACS, a nationally renowned authority on surgical weight-loss procedures and a leader in the rapidly evolving field of Bariatric surgery shares the most current, unbiased information available on the revolutionary weight-loss treatments. He provides those considering outpatient weight-loss surgery a detailed, comprehensive, compassionate guide to choosing, undergoing, and living well after such a procedure. Written in clear, direct, easy-to-follow language and containing real-life personal stories, educational illustrations, and a comprehensive resource section, Dr. Sasse presents an invaluable resource for the medical community and anyone considering a Bariatric surgical procedure today. Outpatient Weight Loss has gained strong endorsements from the medical community and a positive review in Library Journal.

Doctor's Orders
101 Medically-Proven Tips for Losing Weight
Kent Sasse MD, MPH, FACS

This simple yet powerful tips resource provides meaningful evidence-based practical and effective tips for initial weight loss and long-term weight maintenance. It touches on key topics that help remind readers to initiate and ingrain long-term healthy behaviors. It points out small meaningful steps that each person can take on the road to a healthier weight. Readers can take advantage of Dr. Sasse's significant insight and reading of the scientific literature to make the weight-loss journey a success.

Life-Changing Weight Loss:
Feel More Energetic and Live a More Active Life with a Medically Based Weight Loss Program
Kent Sasse MD, MPH, FACS

Combining the science of weight loss with inspiration and advice that has dramatically improved the lives of many people, this guide offers a compelling case that change is possible and that losing weight may be the most important life change a person can make. Dr. Kent Sasse, the renowned founder of iMetabolic, a nationally recognized, state-of-the-art weight-loss institute, successfully brings together psychologists, personal trainers, physicians, life coaches, registered dietitians, and support groups to show you how.

Shakin' it Up
by Chef Dave Fouts with Nutritional Consultation by Vicki Bovee, M.S., R.D.

This recipe book delivers wonderful and creative shake recipes from a trained chef who has undergone Bariatric surgery himself and understands the need for diversity and flavor during these very important phases before and after surgery. In addition, this book is valuable to anyone making meal replacements a normal part of their weight loss and weight maintenance routines.

Smooth Foods
by Chef Dave Fouts with Nutritional Consultation by Vicki Bovee, M.S., R.D.

This recipe book focuses on the second eating phase after weight loss surgery, when smooth, easy-to-digest foods are the order of the day. Chef Dave Fouts provides recipes geared toward providing variety with sound nutrition while still focusing on the protein, vitamin, and texture needs of anyone who has undergone weight-loss surgery.

Soft Foods
by Chef Dave Fouts with Nutritional Consultation by Vicki Bovee, M.S., R.D.

This recipe book focuses on the third eating phase after weight loss surgery, when soft foods, become the order of the day. Soft Foods is the final connection before the introduction of regular foods back into the patient's routine. Chef Dave Fouts provides recipes geared toward providing variety with sound nutrition while still focusing on the protein, vitamin, and texture needs of anyone who has undergone weight-loss surgery. In reality, many of these recipes can be utilized during the regular course of one's routine as they are healthy and nutritious for the whole family.

E-Books

Adolescents and Weight-Loss Surgery: The Benefits and Risks

After Weight Loss Surgery: The Keys to Weight-Loss Success After Bariatric Surgery

Seniors and Weight-Loss Surgery: The Benefits and Risks

Which Weight-Loss Procedure Is Right For Me?: The Latest Data on Bariatric Surgery Helps You Decide

Notes